NATIONAL COOPERATIVE HIGHWAY RESEARCH PROGRAM

NCHRP RESEARCH REPORT 1111

BEHAVIORAL TRAFFIC SAFETY COOPERATIVE RESEARCH PROGRAM

BTSCRP RESEARCH REPORT 12

Diagnostic Assessment and Countermeasure Selection
A TOOLBOX FOR TRAFFIC SAFETY PRACTITIONERS

John L. Campbell
Liberty Hoekstra-Atwood
EXPONENT
Bellevue, WA

Chris Monk
EXPONENT
Washington, DC

Audra K. Fraser
EXPONENT
Irvine, CA

Darren J. Torbic
Ingrid B. Potts
TEXAS A&M UNIVERSITY
TEXAS TRANSPORTATION INSTITUTE
College Station, TX

T0295438

Subscriber Categories
Highways • Operations and Traffic Management • Safety and Human Factors

Research sponsored by the American Association of State Highway and Transportation Officials
in cooperation with the Federal Highway Administration and under the direction and
oversight of the Governors Highway Safety Association

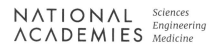

NATIONAL ACADEMIES *Sciences Engineering Medicine*

TRB TRANSPORTATION RESEARCH BOARD

2024

NATIONAL COOPERATIVE HIGHWAY RESEARCH PROGRAM

Systematic, well-designed, and implementable research is the most effective way to solve many problems facing state departments of transportation (DOTs) administrators and engineers. Often, highway problems are of local or regional interest and can best be studied by state DOTs individually or in cooperation with their state universities and others. However, the accelerating growth of highway transportation results in increasingly complex problems of wide interest to highway authorities. These problems are best studied through a coordinated program of cooperative research.

Recognizing this need, the leadership of the American Association of State Highway and Transportation Officials (AASHTO) in 1962 initiated an objective national highway research program using modern scientific techniques—the National Cooperative Highway Research Program (NCHRP). NCHRP is supported on a continuing basis by funds from participating member states of AASHTO and receives the full cooperation and support of the Federal Highway Administration (FHWA), United States Department of Transportation, under Agreement No. 693JJ31950003.

The Transportation Research Board (TRB) of the National Academies of Sciences, Engineering, and Medicine was requested by AASHTO to administer the research program because of TRB's recognized objectivity and understanding of modern research practices. TRB is uniquely suited for this purpose for many reasons: TRB maintains an extensive committee structure from which authorities on any highway transportation subject may be drawn; TRB possesses avenues of communications and cooperation with federal, state, and local governmental agencies, universities, and industry; TRB's relationship to the National Academies is an insurance of objectivity; and TRB maintains a full-time staff of specialists in highway transportation matters to bring the findings of research directly to those in a position to use them.

The program is developed on the basis of research needs identified by chief administrators and other staff of the highway and transportation departments, by committees of AASHTO, and by the FHWA. Topics of the highest merit are selected by the AASHTO Special Committee on Research and Innovation (R&I), and each year R&I's recommendations are proposed to the AASHTO Board of Directors and the National Academies. Research projects to address these topics are defined by NCHRP, and qualified research agencies are selected from submitted proposals. Administration and surveillance of research contracts are the responsibilities of the National Academies and TRB.

The needs for highway research are many, and NCHRP can make significant contributions to solving highway transportation problems of mutual concern to many responsible groups. The program, however, is intended to complement, rather than to substitute for or duplicate, other highway research programs.

NCHRP RESEARCH REPORT 1111

Project 22-45
ISSN 2572-3766 (Print)
ISSN 2572-3774 (Online)
ISBN 978-0-309-70997-2
Library of Congress Control Number 2024940434

Published research reports of the

NATIONAL COOPERATIVE HIGHWAY RESEARCH PROGRAM

are available from

National Academies Press
500 Fifth Street, NW, Keck 360
Washington, DC 20001

(800) 624-6242

and can be ordered through the Internet by going to

https://nap.nationalacademies.org

Printed in the United States of America

BEHAVIORAL TRAFFIC SAFETY COOPERATIVE RESEARCH PROGRAM

Since the widespread introduction of motor vehicles more than a century ago, crashes involving their operation remain a significant public health concern. While there have been enormous improvements in highway design and construction, as well as motor vehicle safety, which have been instrumental in lowering the rate of crashes per million miles in the United States, more than 35,000 people die every year in motor vehicle crashes. In far too many cases, the root causes of the crashes are the unsafe behaviors of motor vehicle operators, cyclists, and pedestrians. Understanding human behaviors and developing effective countermeasures to unsafe ones is difficult and remains a major weakness in our traffic safety efforts.

The Behavioral Traffic Safety Cooperative Research Program (BTSCRP) develops practical solutions to save lives, prevent injuries, and reduce costs of road traffic crashes associated with unsafe behaviors. BTSCRP is a forum for coordinated and collaborative research efforts. It is managed by the Transportation Research Board (TRB) under the direction and oversight of the Governors Highway Safety Association (GHSA) with funding provided by the National Highway Traffic Safety Administration (NHTSA). Funding for the program was originally established in Moving Ahead for Progress in the 21st Century (MAP-21), Subsection 402(c), which created the National Cooperative Research and Evaluation Program (NCREP). Fixing America's Surface Transportation (FAST) Act continued the program. In 2017, GHSA entered into an agreement with TRB to manage the research activities, with the program name changed to Behavioral Traffic Safety Cooperative Research Program. The GHSA Executive Board serves as the governing board for the BTSCRP. The Board consists of officers, representatives of the 10 NHTSA regions, and committee and task force chairs. The Research Committee Chair appoints committee members who recommend projects for funding and provide oversight for the activities of BTSCRP. Its ultimate goal is to oversee a quality research program that is committed to addressing research issues facing State Highway Safety Offices. The Executive Board meets annually to approve research projects. Each selected project is assigned to a panel, appointed by TRB, which provides technical guidance and counsel throughout the life of the project. The majority of panel members represent the intended users of the research projects and have an important role in helping to implement the results. BTSCRP produces a series of research reports and other products such as guidebooks for practitioners. Primary emphasis is placed on disseminating BTSCRP results to the intended users of the research: State Highway Safety Offices and their constituents.

BTSCRP RESEARCH REPORT 12

Project BTS-14
ISSN 2766-5976 (Print)
ISSN 2766-5984 (Online)
ISBN 978-0-309-70997-2
Library of Congress Control Number 2024940434

Published research reports of the

BEHAVIORAL TRAFFIC SAFETY COOPERATIVE RESEARCH PROGRAM

are available from

National Academies Press
500 Fifth Street, NW, Keck 360
Washington, DC 20001

(800) 624-6242

and can be ordered through the Internet by going to

https://nap.nationalacademies.org

Printed in the United States of America

NATIONAL ACADEMIES
Sciences
Engineering
Medicine

COOPERATIVE RESEARCH PROGRAMS

CRP STAFF FOR NCHRP RESEARCH REPORT 1111/ BTSCRP RESEARCH REPORT 12

Waseem Dekelbab, *Deputy Director, Cooperative Research Programs, and Manager, National Cooperative Highway Research Program*
Richard A. Retting, *Senior Program Officer*
Dajaih Bias-Johnson, *Senior Program Assistant*
Natalie Barnes, *Director of Publications*
Heather DiAngelis, *Associate Director of Publications*

NCHRP PROJECT 22-45/BTSCRP PROJECT BTS-14 PANEL
Field of Design—Area of Vehicle Barrier Systems

Priyanka Alluri, *Florida International University, Miami, FL*
John C. Milton, *Washington State Department of Transportation, Olympia, WA*
Sung Yoon Park, *Maryland State Highway Administration, Hanover, MD*
Bernadette Estioko Phelan, *Phelan International LLC, Scottsdale, AZ*
Robert A. Skehan, *Maine Department of Transportation, Augusta, ME*
John S. Tomlinson, *Idaho Transportation Department, Boise, ID*
Christopher J. Turner, *Kansas Third District Judicial Court, Topeka, KS*
Dustin R. Witt, *South Dakota Department of Transportation, Pierre, SD*
Jonathan S. Wood, *Iowa State University, Ames, IA*
Karen Scurry, *FHWA Liaison*
Derek A. Troyer, *FHWA Liaison*
Kelly K. Hardy, *AASHTO Liaison*
Bernardo B. Kleiner, *TRB Liaison*

AUTHOR ACKNOWLEDGMENTS

The research reported herein was performed under NCHRP Project 22-45/BTSCRP Project BTS-14 by Exponent, with the Texas Transportation Institute (TTI) of Texas A&M University serving as a research partner.

By Richard A. Retting
Staff Officer
Transportation Research Board

NCHRP Research Report 1111/BTSCRP Research Report 12 presents a toolbox to help highway safety practitioners diagnose contributing factors leading to crashes for use in selecting appropriate countermeasures. To develop this toolbox, the research team conducted a systematic literature review; developed comprehensive evaluation and analysis procedures, methods, and tools; and conducted a workshop to demonstrate the use of the draft toolbox to receive feedback from practitioners. This publication will be of interest to state departments of transportation and other stakeholders concerned with diagnosing contributing factors leading to crashes for use in selecting appropriate countermeasures.

Successful safety management practices require a thorough understanding of factors contributing to motor vehicle crashes. Continuous advancements in data-driven safety analysis, as well as the countermeasures and technologies available to address crashes, create challenges in maintaining a safety workforce proficient in the state of the practice. In many cases, agencies continue to use approaches such as descriptive statistics and anecdotal information to perform the diagnostic assessment without a thorough understanding of the expectations for a given context or road type. Additionally, choosing an effective countermeasure requires an examination of the human factors, behavioral factors, future development, prevailing or predicted crash types, and mix of road users to determine the most appropriate treatments to apply. Doing so allows the selected countermeasure to reduce crashes to the greatest extent possible. However, in many cases, practitioners have limited understanding of the potential for a treatment selection to affect other road users. A better understanding of these relationships and trade-offs could inform design choices and ultimately result in safer roadways for all road users.

Under NCHRP Project 22-45/BTSCRP Project BTS-14, Exponent was asked to develop a toolbox for diagnosing contributing factors leading to crashes that will aid practitioners in selecting appropriate countermeasures in modally diverse contexts. The research team (1) performed a detailed review and assessment of the research literature related to crash diagnosis, factors leading to crashes, and countermeasure selection; (2) developed comprehensive evaluation and analysis procedures, methods, and tools to support understanding and analysis of crash contributing factors; (3) conducted a workshop to demonstrate the use of the new and/or enhanced methods and tools, and to receive feedback from practitioners; and (4) developed a toolbox to help highway safety practitioners diagnose contributing factors leading to crashes for use in selecting appropriate countermeasures.

In addition to this report, the following deliverables are available on the National Academies Press website (nap.nationalacademies.org) by searching for *NCHRP Research Report 1111/ BTSCRP Research Report 12*:

- A technical memorandum on implementation of research findings and products,
- A PowerPoint presentation, and
- A conduct of research report.

CONTENTS

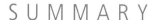

Diagnostic Assessment and Countermeasure Selection: A Toolbox for Traffic Safety Practitioners

Purpose. A Toolbox for Traffic Safety Practitioners provides new tools for diagnosing the contributing factors to crashes and then selecting appropriate countermeasures. It addresses a wide variety of contributing factors to crashes to further practitioners' understanding of how to balance trade-off decisions that must be made concerning both diagnostic assessments and countermeasure selection. Key goals of this toolbox are to (1) support robust and comprehensive assessments of crashes and subsequent implementation of effective countermeasures and (2) advance the design and operation of roadways that are predictable, support the visibility and conspicuity of key elements, avoid strong demands, and provide all road users enough time to react to the full range of driving situations and conditions.

How to use this toolbox. This toolbox is intended to help those who diagnose contributing crash factors identify and select effective countermeasures for these crashes. The reader can use Chapters 2–9 of this toolbox for search-and-find activities to obtain (1) background knowledge that can further their understanding of key concepts and related research and concepts and (2) practical tools that identify key concepts and questions that can frame and guide the diagnostics process. Chapter 10 contains step-by-step decision trees to aid in countermeasure selection for a broad range of facility types and crash types. Chapter 11 provides a set of techniques and tools that can help practitioners assess roadway design and operations and identify elements that impose a high demand on drivers. Figures, tables, and examples are shared throughout the text to illustrate concepts, present data, and provide templates for practitioner use. Some of these materials appear in more than one chapter to facilitate usage of the varied tools.

This toolbox is intended for use by a variety of traffic safety practitioners, including planners, designers, engineers, and safety analysts. Planners and designers can use it to make initial estimates of the demands that a future facility might place on road users, in terms of high-level topics like meeting expectations and visibility (e.g., sight distance and planned lighting), as well as topics like the complexity of traffic control devices (i.e., workload). Engineers can use it to assess these topics from an operations perspective, as well as to assess more detailed topics like available perception-response times based on features such as signal timing and use scenarios involving mixed modalities (e.g., motor vehicles and bicycles). Safety analysts can use it to assess actual safety performance (i.e., crash frequency and severity), including enforcement records (e.g., speeding violations), tort claims (i.e., evaluations of individual crashes), and groups of similar crashes at the same roadway location (i.e., "hot spots").

The role of human error in roadway crashes. Several broad, in-depth studies (e.g., Treat et al., 1979; Wierwille et al., 2002; Singh, 2015, and Dong and Wood, 2023) have examined roadway crashes and have found that some form of human error is a key contributor to most crashes. The types of errors humans commit vary; they can include failing to perceive and recognize a hazardous situation, making bad decisions, or making an error in driver performance. All road users have a limited capacity to receive and process information from the environment; thus, inattention and distraction are frequent contributors to crashes. Also important to a proper understanding of the nature of crashes is to avoid attributing most crashes to a single contributing factor—crashes often have more than one contributing factor (Dingus et al., 2006). An effective framework and methodology for the diagnostic assessment of crashes should include not just a review and analysis of relevant road user, environmental, and vehicle factors, but also the interactions among these factors. Chapter 2 includes a broader discussion of the contributing factors to roadway crashes.

Driver errors can reflect aberrant driver behaviors or human factors issues. While most crashes reflect some sort of driver error, some of these errors (approximately 57%) reflect aberrant driver behavior issues such as impaired driving because of drugs or alcohol, road rage, fatigue, or distraction/inattention, while others (approximately 30%) reflect human factors issues, that is, roadway designs and traffic operation features that place demands on road users that may exceed their capabilities. This distinction between human factors issues and aberrant driver behavior issues is crucial, as they reflect different contributing factors to crashes and corresponding differences in effective countermeasures. Human factors issues include contributing factors to crashes that generally reflect mismatches between the demands placed on the road user by roadway design and traffic engineering features and the inherent physical, perceptual, and cognitive capabilities and limitations of road users. Thus, crashes related to human factors issues may be addressed through some change in the roadway environment (Campbell et al., 2012).

Aberrant driver behavior issues, however, include contributing factors to crashes that generally reflect deliberate violations of law or unsafe driving practices, such as texting while driving, inattention, or driving while impaired by alcohol. Such issues are generally best addressed through behavioral strategies such as training, regulations, or enforcement (Venkatraman et al., 2021). Chapter 4 summarizes research relevant to this topic and provides a diagnostic process to help practitioners distinguish between crashes that primarily reflect human factors issues from those that reflect aberrant driver behaviors.

Roadways are a communications device and are always communicating to road users. A helpful principle provided by the positive guidance approach to design (Lunenfeld and Alexander, 1990; Russell, 1998) is for designers and engineers to consider the highway system as a holistic source of information—a real-time communications device—that is continuously sampled by road users for meaningful information. Critically, roadways are always sending messages to the road user; the key for the practitioner is to design, operate, and continuously evaluate the roadway so that the right messages are consistently provided at the right time to support timely and effective road user behaviors.

A framework for thinking about crashes: roadway demands versus road-user capabilities. Whether human factors issues, aberrant driver behaviors, or some other factors are the culprit, many crashes reflect a fairly simple calculation: crashes are more likely to happen when the demands of the roadway environment exceed the capabilities of the roadway user. In particular, driving requires a complex series of physical actions and mental operations that vary considerably across driving contexts, situations, and conditions. While different driving situations and conditions place different demands on the driver (e.g., making a left turn at an unsignalized intersection against traffic versus driving on an interstate in light traffic), all driving situations require that drivers remain alert and attentive.

Trade-offs in a multimodal transportation network. Trade-offs refer to the inevitable give and take around balancing multiple safety options, including assessments of the strengths and weaknesses associated with safety considerations for all road users; that is, drivers, pedestrians, bicyclists, and transit users. Both the diagnostic assessment process and the countermeasure selection process should include the compromises, balance, and perhaps exchange between desirable but incompatible elements that characterize making decisions about roadway safety. Diagnostic assessment includes a recognition that road users themselves make trade-offs all the time between convenience, safety, travel time, and costs and that crash assessments should take this into consideration. Countermeasure selection by the safety professional should include trade-offs between key variables, including countermeasure efficacy, specific safety benefits, unanticipated outcomes, and feasibility (e.g., time and cost).

Importance of evaluation. Critical to improving safety performance (i.e., crash frequency and severity) is the evaluation (a fifth "E" that can be added to the four "E's" of highway safety—engineering, education, enforcement, and emergency medical services) of crash data in modal and facility contexts to assess crashes and aid the selection and design of counter-measures. While program evaluation might be considered something to worry about after countermeasures have been identified, this fifth "E" should be implemented at every stage of the safety improvement process and include input and involvement from the range of transportation professionals involved, including planners, designers, engineers, and safety analysts. In short, having an evaluative mindset throughout the crash prevention process can add rigor and purpose to safety improvement planning. Several chapters of this toolbox discuss the importance of evaluation throughout the diagnostic assessment and counter-measure selection process and include tools and methods for conducting evaluations, especially Chapters 3 and 9.

Diagnostic Assessment in the Safe System

Overview of the Safe System approach. The Safe System approach seeks to plan, design, and operate a road system that recognizes that humans make mistakes, have limited physiological abilities to safely negotiate complex situations, and have a limited tolerance of kinetic energy forces (Signor et al., 2018; Welle et al., 2018; Finkel et al., 2020). A key goal of this holistic approach is to create a system that reduces the risk of kinetic energy transfer occurring in the first place and reduces the amount of energy transfer in the event of a crash to an amount that can be tolerated by humans. Overall, the Safe System approach incorporates five elements: safe road users, safe vehicles, safe speeds, safe roads, and post-crash care. The diagnostic process should very much be considered to be an evaluative activity, as the fifth "E" (evaluation) should exist at every stage of the safety management process and not just toward the end of the process as part of countermeasure evaluation. The approach includes the five "E's" of traffic safety but also encompasses planners, designers, operators, and users of the trans-portation system to prevent fatal crashes and reduce crash severity.

A general process for diagnostic assessment. A diagnostic assessment process that incor-porates the holistic elements associated with Safe System will explicitly incorporate general consideration of all road users but also

- Consider pre-, during-, and post-crash factors that might have contributed to the crash itself, as well as post-crash survivability;
- Evaluate specific issues related to the role of perception-response time, expectations, visibility, and workload/demand; and
- Produce a detailed summary of possible contributing factors and their likely interactions.

Figure 1 summarizes a process for diagnostic assessment and emphasizes the importance of considering not just crash and site data but also key human factors issues (discussed in more detail in this summary and in Chapters 5–8) that are often the key contributing factors

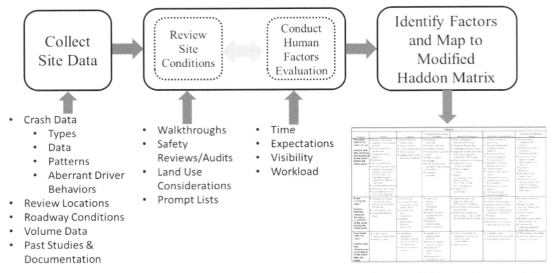

Consider pre-, during-, and post-crash factors

Figure 1.   A general process for diagnostic assessment in the Safe System.

to crashes. It will also be useful to incorporate aberrant driver behaviors (such as impaired or distracted driving) into the analysis.

The focus at this stage of the diagnostic assessment process is on thinking like a virtual road user and identifying and understanding the roadway components that could contribute to confusion, poor visibility, misperceptions, high workload, distraction, or other potential road user errors at a particular site. Solutions in the form of countermeasures or treatments (discussed in Chapters 9 and 10) are not sought at this stage of crash evaluations.

Figure 1 includes a step to develop a Modified Haddon Matrix as part of the diagnostic assessment process. Haddon's epidemiological view of injury (Haddon, 1972; National Committee for Injury Prevention and Control, 1989) outlines three phases to crash evaluations:

1. A pre-crash phase that includes those factors that influence whether a crash will occur and then result in injuries
2. A crash event phase that includes those factors that influence injury severity during the crash event
3. A post-crash phase that includes those factors that influence the survivability of the crash after the event

To augment this approach, John Milton and Ida van Schalkwyk of the Washington State Department of Transportation (personal communication, January 17, 2022) have developed a framework that directly considers all road users (e.g., the volume of biking and walking) and supports the social safety environment. Consistent with the Safe System approach, it has also added user-mix considerations and interactions between these factors. Table 1 shows a Modified Haddon Matrix applied to motor vehicle crashes in the Safe System. This matrix was developed by Milton and van Schalkwyk and is used with their kind permission.

By introducing social environment factors, safety professionals are asked to consider the implications of attitudes, biases, and equity decision-making frameworks for humans operating in the roadway environment. Doing so expands the potential diagnostic assessments that safety professionals perform.

Table 1. Modified Haddon Matrix applied to motor vehicle crashes in the Safe System.

Phases	Factors					
	Human	Vehicle	Physical Environment/ Context	Social Environment	User-Mix Considerations	Interactions Between Users
Pre-event *(Before the crash occurs)* **Factors that may increase the likelihood of the crash before the crash event**	• Driver's perceptual, cognitive, and physical abilities • Alcohol and drug impairment • Impairment from fatigue • Distraction • Driver experience • Ability to perceive and react to unexpected events in a driving environment (e.g., understanding the potential for different road users) • Alertness/attentiveness • Familiarity with route • Expectations for the environment/facility	• Maintenance of brakes, tires • Speed of travel • Load characteristics • Size of vehicle • Safety and/or driver assistance features • Type of vehicle (e.g., commercial vehicle, passenger vehicle, motorcycle, bicycle, scooter)	• Roadway markings • Divided highways • Roadway lighting • Intersection type and angle • Road curvature • Signage • Walking and biking availability, facility type, separation • Roadway shoulders • Ambient and vehicle lighting	• Public attitudes on drinking and driving • Impaired driving laws • Graduated licensing laws • Seat belt, helmet, and other personal protective equipment laws • Risky behavior prominence • Support for injury prevention efforts • Positive safety culture • Equity considerations for lower income (e.g., PPE, driver ed., scholarships) • Presence of passengers	• Volume of walking and biking • Type and separation of path/shoulder sidewalk • Route directness • Crossing distance from generators • Reliance on transit, walking, and biking • Lighting Scale • Sense of security of routes • Intersection turning speeds and priorities for operations • Mid-block crossing controls • Intersection type • Speed management	• Speed setting consistent with user mix • Ability to maintain consistent operating speeds • Choice-making based on road users' safety and security • Common behaviors • Education and enforcement • Ability to turn on red, permitted, and protected signals for vulnerable road users (VRUs) • Access management
Event *(During the crash)* **Factors that may influence the injury or severity of the crash during the crash event**	• Spread out energy in time and space with seat belt and/or airbag use • Child restraint use • Personal protective gear	• Vehicle size (also consider mass and center of gravity) • Crashworthiness of vehicle, overall safety rating • Airbags (type and placement) • Padded dashboards and steering wheel	• Guard rails, median barriers, breakaway devices • Presence of fixed objects near the roadway • Roadside embankments • Other road users	• Seat belt, child restraint, and other PPE laws are followed. • Enforcement of occupant restraint laws • Motorcycle and bicycle helmet laws or use, or both are followed and accepted	• Travel speeds • Vehicle size and type • Design exposure that tends to increase speed or threats during crossing or walking on facilities • Separation of users • Proximity of VRUs to vehicles	• Speeds resulting in injury • Angle of crash through design and operation • Vision, speed judgment • Protective equipment and restraint use • Crash-worthy roadside hardware and clear zone
Post-event *(After the crash)* **Factors that may influence the survivability of the crash after the event**	• Crash victim's general health status • Age of victims	• Gas tanks designed to maintain integrity during a crash to minimize fires • Ability to extract injured • Vehicle size, mass, and center of gravity	• Availability of effective emergency medical services (EMS) systems • Ability to respond quickly to crash • Distance to trauma care • Rehabilitation programs in place	• Public support for an emergency, trauma care, and post-crash rehabilitation • EMS training	• Trauma center availability and proximity • Emergency response	• Redundancy of system • Ability to respond and transport to care

This modification of the original Haddon Matrix aims to present a framework that more directly considers all road users and the supporting social safety environment. It is best to generate a Modified Haddon Matrix that includes all possible factors impacting safety performance (crash frequency and severity). Specifically, the Matrix should include any factors and combinations of factors (interactions) that could reasonably contribute to the known or suspected opportunities for reducing crash potentials at the site under investigation. Broad considerations should include crash or conflict type, frequency, severity, and contributing factors, as well as on-the-scene observations of the facility and representative traffic movements (including pedestrians, bicyclists, and transit vehicles). In this regard, some interactions may be quantitative and specific, while others may be qualitative and reflect possible impacts.

Chapter 3 presents a more detailed discussion of diagnostic assessment in the Safe System.

Evaluating the role of human factors issues in crash diagnostics. Treat et al. (1979) and several subsequent large-scale crash studies have shown that, while most crashes indeed reflect some form of driver error, a subset of these errors (approximately 57%) reflect primarily "driver-only" issues such as impaired driving because of drugs or alcohol, road issues (including roadway designs) and traffic operation features place demands on road users that may exceed their capabilities (i.e., human factors issues). Human factors issues, then, are simply interactions between the roadway and the road user that contribute to crashes.

While a thorough review of human factors is beyond the scope of this toolbox, decades of crash analyses and studies of driver behavior and performance (Wierwille et al., 2002; Campbell et al., 2012; Theeuwes and van der Horst, 2012; Permanent International Association of Road Congresses [PIARC], 2019a) make clear that the following four human factors issues are key to the efficacy of roadways as communication devices and the general safety performance (i.e., crash frequency and severity) of roadways:

Perception-response time (PRT)—A common thread in the circumstances that lead to many roadway crashes is time, specifically, a lack of time for the driver (for example) to respond to an upcoming object in the roadway, a change in roadway characteristics or a navigation demand. PRT is comprised of multiple components that generally overlap in time and includes the time to detect a target, process the information, decide on a response, and initiate a reaction. The other key human factors issues—expectations, visibility, and workload—primarily present challenges to a driver because of the time constraints imposed by the driving task. A large body of research involving laboratory and on-road studies has helped estimate approximate driver PRT values under a variety of situations. Although this range is wide (roughly 0.5 to 2.5 seconds), the data on PRTs can have significant utility in crash diagnostics and roadway design. The "Green Book" (American Association of State Highway and Transportation Officials [AASHTO], 2018) recommends a design criterion of 2.5 seconds to include the capabilities of most drivers under most highway conditions, but actual PRTs will be situation dependent. Specifically, driver PRTs will be determined by several factors, including driver expectations, driver age, the conspicuity of detected roadway objects, and vehicle speed.

In a crash sequence, vehicle speed translates directly into the time available for drivers to react; the time issue therefore highlights the importance of posted speed selection by designers and the speed choices made by drivers. Perhaps one of the most direct ways that roadway designers can improve safety performance (i.e., crash frequency and severity) is to design the roadway and accompanying operations to give more time for road users to perceive, decide on a response to, and react to situations and conditions.

Expectations—Drivers rely on their general knowledge and past experience driving a particular facility to aid the continuous driving task and manage new information they need to process. Designing roadway environments in accordance with driver expectations is a crucial way to accommodate a road user's inherent human limitations and make the roadway predictable for road users. The idea of predictability in design is key, as basic facility design and related traffic operations should avoid surprising road users. Predictability is the key benefit to meeting users' expectations; predictability allows the road user to place a roadway into a predefined category that—in turn—dictates behavior. In this regard, roadways that meet user expectations can function like a familiar "script" that directs and supports behaviors that are both effective and timely. Navigating the roadways as a driver, bicyclist, or pedestrian benefits from physical environments, sequences of required actions, and interactions with others that are predictable. Expectations are central to how a driver monitors, perceives, and interprets the roadway environment, makes decisions, and then acts or responds. Variances from driver expectations are a key source of misperceived and misinterpreted information, slowed response times, and driver errors.

For the driver, expectations are closely related to the broader principle of design consistency. Design consistency is one of the most basic principles in human factors and system design. Consistency improves user performance because it facilitates the user's ability to predict what the system will do in any given situation; it provides rules that govern relationships between elements in the environment (e.g., signage and geometry) and driver responses (e.g., navigation and speed selection). The same underlying principle applies to other road users, such as bicyclists, pedestrians, and transit users.

Visibility—Visibility refers to the quality or state of being visible and relates to concepts such as conspicuity and sight distance. Approximately 90% of the information used by a driver is obtained visually (Hills, 1980) and, according to Treat et al. (1979), one of the leading environmental factors related to traffic crashes is visibility. Visibility is closely related to conspicuity, defined by Krauss (2015) as "those characteristics of an object or condition that determine the likelihood that it will come to the attention of an observer" (p. 57). In other words, conspicuity refers to how noticeable or visible an object is.

A driver's ability to select and act on even highly visible and conspicuous objects may be impacted by the amount and type of competing stimuli (e.g., pedestrians, other vehicles, signs, markings, buildings, or planters) in the immediate environment (Edquist and Johnston, 2008). Thus, the complexity and clutter associated with a visual scene impact visibility. Drivers' visibility may be reduced because of physical limitations, such as inclement weather conditions (e.g., fog, rain, snow, or sun glare), vehicle conditions (e.g., burned-out headlights or a dirty windshield), the geometry of the roadway, and other scene elements. Regarding perceptual or cognitive limitations, visibility may also be impacted by driver distraction or inattention, diminished visual acuity, or reduced contrast sensitivity (Hills, 1980).

In general, road signs, lane markings, and lighting are roadway-design elements that can significantly impact visibility, especially at night (FHWA, 2022a), and help address visibility limitations based on roadway geometry (e.g., sharp horizontal curves or vertical curves). For example, advance signage can inform the driver of upcoming limited visibility situations, and well-maintained retroreflective signs can improve nighttime visibility and reduce the risk of crashes by making signs appear brighter and easier to see and read from a distance. Similarly, well-maintained lane markings can make road curvatures more visible from a greater distance, thereby preparing the driver for unexpected curves. Finally, roadway lighting helps make roadways, surrounding areas, and road users, such as pedestrians, more visible at night.

Task demand/Workload—Workload refers to the overall demands placed on an individual by a particular activity, including effort, task complexity, time usage, and the nature of possible interference between concurrent tasks (Gartner and Murphy, 1979; Gawron, 2000; Angell et al., 2006). The workload in the driving context generally refers to the demands placed on an individual while performing driving tasks, which can be impacted by driver effort, task complexity, time constraints, and potential interference among multiple concurrent tasks (Tijerina et al., 1996). A useful shorthand for thinking about workload is to consider the time available to complete a task relative to the specific demands of the task; in other words, workload = time/task. While effort and time pressures are key aspects of workload, in the driving domain, workload is frequently described in terms of the following (Richard et al., 2006):

- Perceptual requirements (e.g., detecting and making sense of what is seen, heard, and felt)
- Decision-making/cognitive needs (e.g., making decisions to go, stop, or turn; integrating what you perceive with things you know, such as rules of the road; or using your previous experience with a roadway facility to help decide what maneuver is appropriate)
- Psychomotor/response needs [e.g., executing a decision, taking an action (such as a driver changing their point of gaze to somewhere else within the visual scene), braking, or changing lanes]

Driving is a demanding activity, as drivers are continuously performing several tasks at the same time, often while moving at a high rate of speed. These tasks include visual scanning of the environment, perception and identification of task-relevant elements (e.g., other vehicles, pedestrians, traffic signs, and traffic signals), lane maintenance, and speed control. Critically, the driving environment is ever-changing, often requiring relatively high vigilance and attention to these tasks. Importantly, workload concerns are not limited to drivers, and the demands placed on other road users should be considered as well. For example, pedestrians crossing a roadway need to plan a path, monitor for hazards such as vehicles and bicycles, and then execute a crossing maneuver. Likewise, bicyclists riding within the lane or on the shoulder of a rural road have to watch the roadway ahead, maintain position within a lane or bike path, and continuously monitor for and avoid in-path objects.

The nature and source of high task demands will vary considerably across different roadway types and driving conditions. Table 2 shows some typical roadway types and highlights features that could increase demands.

Chapters 5 through 8 in the toolbox provide more comprehensive discussions of these four human factors issues, including questions for each that can be used as part of the diagnostic assessment process presented in Figure 1. Quantifying workload/demand for drivers requires conducting workload analysis for a given roadway segment and driving task, and Chapter 11 provides a set of techniques and tools that can help practitioners assess roadway design and operations and identify elements that impose a high demand on drivers. These methods aim to consider what a roadway requires of drivers and include ways to assess the number of static and dynamic elements that require the driver's attention, comprehension, decisions, and potential action, as well as more involved workload assessment techniques.

Selecting Effective Countermeasures

Effective countermeasures decrease the demands placed on the road user and/or augment the road user's capabilities in some fashion. Roadways are communication devices, and they are at all times communicating a host of messages to the road user. Sometimes these messages are helpful and intended by the roadway designer, and sometimes not. Countermeasures provide an opportunity to improve how the roadway designer communicates with the road user and can decrease the crash frequency or severity at a particular site. Once again, many crashes happen when the demands of the roadway environment exceed the capabilities of the roadway user. In this regard, it is important to recognize that roadway countermeasures

Table 2. Roadway types and elements that can increase demands on road users (photos by Samuel Tignor, 2021; used with permission).

Roadway Types	Elements That Can Increase Demands on Road Users
Interstate Highways 	• High speeds can translate into reduced time to respond to conflicting vehicles. • High levels of visual demand, including frequent glances to adjacent lanes, are required to respond to multi-vehicle moving hazards (e.g., merge maneuvers, cut-ins, and stopped vehicles ahead). • Conflicting moving vehicles could enter the road from the ramp. • Perceptual and decision-making demand is higher with smaller gaps (dense traffic) for merging and lane changing.
State Routes 	• Curves and vegetation obstruct delineation cues and oncoming vehicles near a hill. • Potential for hidden driveways • Visibility/expectancy at intersections • Presence of bicyclists and pedestrians • Visibility/expectancy is questionable at unexpected intersections. • Possible conflicts at the crest of a hill and turning road • Guardrail close to roadway restricts possible escape path.
Rural Roads 	• Potential vehicles, pedestrians, or bikes at or beyond the crest • Narrow lane widths on each side of the road • Potential for hidden driveways • Narrow roadway with no centerline plus narrow shoulders • An unexpected vehicle can enter the road from a driveway.
Urban 	• Highly dynamic traffic elements—stopping and turning vehicles, many bicycles, scooters, and pedestrians—are cramped into the intersection. • Challenging road user guidance and navigation in a dense-visual environment • Visibility of other road users (e.g., the two bike lanes in the center of the street are hard to perceive, and pedestrians may be blocked by other vehicles). • Two-way traffic on a cross street • Traffic signals and signs must be perceived and comprehended.
City Center 	• A mix of road users—pedestrians, bicyclists, scooters—often in unexpected locations • Many traffic control devices—traffic signals, signs • Dynamic traffic elements—stopping and turning vehicles • Challenging road user guidance and navigation in a dense-visual environment • Extremely limited visibility/expectancy throughout the street • Large trucks and buses block users' visibility and mobility. • Traffic signals, signs, and pavement markings are blocked by queued vehicles. • User workload is extremely high for all modal users.

operate within this demand versus capabilities framework. Specifically, effective counter-measures decrease the demands placed on the road user and/or augment the road user's capabilities in some fashion. Accordingly, countermeasures should be selected in a manner that links their features and benefits to the underlying contributing factors and human factors issues observed within the crash data or the facility itself.

A countermeasure selection process. This chapter's discussion regarding the counter-measure identification and selection process picks up where the diagnostic assessment process (as illustrated in Figure 1) ended—with a partially completed Modified Haddon Matrix. Figure 2 illustrates the countermeasure identification and selection process and is primarily intended to emphasize the importance of linking countermeasure identification and selection to specific human factors issues (as well as driver behavior issues) identified during the diagnostics process.

The features and benefits of specific countermeasures should be matched to the underlying crash-contributing factors observed within the facility. As an illustration of the need to link countermeasure features with underlying contributing factors to crashes, consider the growing issue of pedestrian fatalities. In 2021, there were 7,388 pedestrians killed in traffic crashes; this reflects a 12.5% increase from 6,565 pedestrian fatalities in 2020 (National Center for Statistics and Analysis [NCSA], 2023a). In 2021, pedestrians accounted for 17% of United States fatalities, up from 14% in 2012. While alcohol is involved in many pedestrian crashes, other characteristics of fatal pedestrian crashes are more closely aligned with human factors issues. For example, 84% occurred in urban areas, 75% occurred outside of intersections, and 77% occurred in the dark. While visibility issues seem obvious from the percentage of pedestrian fatalities occurring in the dark, the fatalities occurring in "outside intersections" locations suggest impacts of expectations—drivers are more likely to anticipate pedestrians near intersections.

Several technology development efforts and safety evaluations have been conducted to help address crashes and fatalities involving pedestrians.

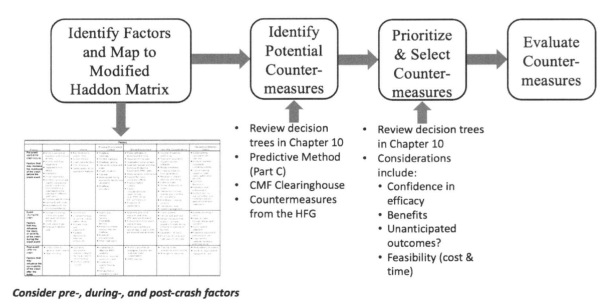

Consider pre-, during-, and post-crash factors

Figure 2. Incorporating the Safe System approach into the countermeasure identification and selection process.

Table 3. Example countermeasures for pedestrian crashes and how they help road users.

Countermeasures	How the Countermeasure Helps Road Users
Advance stop and yield lines	Provides improved visibility of pedestrians for drivers and more time to perceive and react to an unexpected pedestrian incursion by increasing the distance from pedestrians at which drivers are required to stop
Curb extension/bulb-out	Provides improved visibility and sight distance for pedestrians and vehicles and reduces vehicle speeds, giving drivers more time to react to an unexpected pedestrian incursion; reduces pedestrian exposure by reducing pedestrian crossing times and distances
Raised median and pedestrian crossing island	Reduces vehicle speeds, providing more time for drivers to perceive and react to an unexpected pedestrian incursion
Reduce corner radius/crossing distance	Provides improved visibility/sight lines for drivers and reduces turning speeds; reduces pedestrian exposure by reducing pedestrian crossing times and distances
Pedestrian hybrid beacon or a rectangular rapid flashing beacon	Alerts drivers to the presence of pedestrians in a crosswalk, providing drivers with advance warning and more time to react to the situation
Right turn on red restrictions	Reduces pedestrian exposure to turning traffic, where line of sight may be blocked or where drivers' attention is divided
Grade-separated crossings (should only be used when the topography makes them convenient for pedestrians or when the roadway to be crossed is truly inaccessible to pedestrians)	Can eliminate pedestrian exposure to vehicle traffic
Upgrade traffic signal to include leading pedestrian intervals or protected pedestrian phases	Reduces opportunities for conflicts as pedestrians cross
Adaptive traffic signal control strategies to address variable demands because of special events, commercial activities or holiday volumes	Traffic signal cycles that can help pedestrians by providing more efficient and effective crossing times

Table 3 (adapted from Brown et al., 2021) highlights some of these countermeasures and explains how they help road users for example, by reducing speeds (thus giving drivers more time to perceive and react to pedestrians) and/or increasing pedestrian visibility and conspicuity.

Decision trees for selecting countermeasures. Chapter 10 of this toolbox provides a series of decision trees to help practitioners select countermeasures to address target crash types and facility types. The decision trees provide a visual framework for decision-making. Practitioners can select from a series of decision trees that lead them through diagnostic questions to help identify countermeasures that could potentially address crash-contributing factors associated with the crash pattern of interest. Selecting countermeasures for potential implementation, matched to underlying contributing factors to target crash types, is expected to reduce crashes to the greatest extent possible.

The approximately 80 distinct decision trees in Chapter 10 address common crash types that occur along rural and urban roadway segments and intersections, including crashes within the following:

- Rural two-lane roadway segments
- Rural multilane undivided roadway segments

- Rural multilane divided roadway segments
- Urban two-lane roadway segments
- Urban multilane undivided roadway segments
- Urban multilane divided roadway segments
- Rural and urban signalized intersections
- Rural and urban unsignalized intersections

The crash types are further categorized according to common crash contributing factors. Through the diagnostic process outlined in Chapter 3 of this toolbox, practitioners should get a sense of the factors contributing to the crash pattern of interest. Then, by reviewing the respective decision trees, following the logic, and responding to the questions, practitioners will be able to identify a list of potential countermeasures for further consideration in the economic appraisal and project prioritization process. The order of countermeasures presented from top to bottom in the decision trees is not intended to signify any type of prioritization for countermeasure selection or implementation. Priority for selection and implementation is to be based on the applicability of the countermeasure to remedy the crash type of interest at the given site, the cost effectiveness of the implementation of the countermeasure, and other factors, such as trade-offs in safety and mobility between all road users.

Prioritizing candidate countermeasures. The user may want to give a countermeasure greater consideration for implementation if (1) the countermeasure was identified for implementation more than once in response to different diagnostic questions or (2) when the same countermeasure was identified for potential implementation in response to different combinations of contexts, crash types, and contributing factors. Even in these situations, the economic appraisal and project prioritization process, following countermeasure selection, will provide additional details to inform decisions regarding prioritization for implementation based on economic performance measures.

Sample decision tree. Figure 3 shows an example of a decision tree from Chapter 10. In this decision tree, the driving context is rural two-lane segments in which road departure crashes (single-vehicle run-off-road/head-on/sideswipe, opposite direction) are occurring under superelevation and possible decrements in the roadway surface conditions. Critically, final countermeasure selection should include trade-offs between key variables, including countermeasure efficacy, specific safety benefits, unanticipated outcomes, and feasibility (e.g., time and cost).

Context:	Rural Two-lane Segments
Crash Type(s):	Roadway Departure Crashes (Single-vehicle Run-off-road / Head-on / Sideswipe, Opposite Direction)
Contributing Factor(s):	Roadway Surface Condition / Superelevation

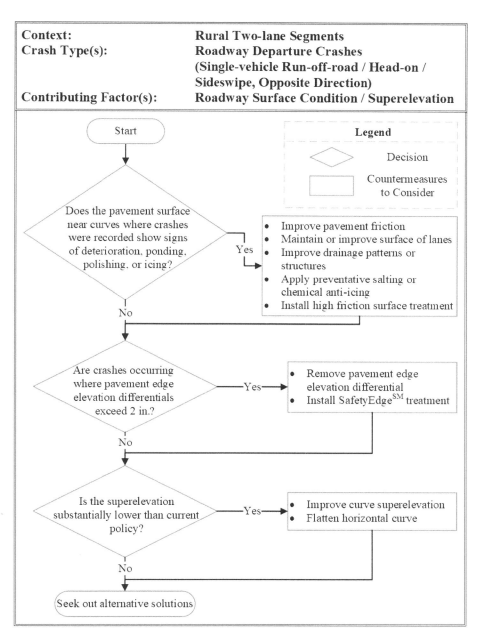

Figure 3. Rural two-lane segments; roadway departure crashes (single-vehicle run-off-road / head-on / sideswipe, opposite direction); roadway surface condition / superelevation.

CHAPTER 1

Introduction

1.1 Background

Successful roadway safety management practices require an understanding of the factors contributing to motor vehicle crashes. Continuous advancements in the science of data-driven safety analysis, as well as in the countermeasures and technologies available to address crashes, create challenges in maintaining a workforce that is proficient in the state of roadway safety management practices. Additionally, choosing an effective countermeasure requires an examination of the human factors, behavioral factors, future development, prevailing or predicted crash types, and mix of road users to determine the most appropriate treatments to apply. Doing so allows the selected countermeasure to be matched to underlying contributing factors, and thereby reduce crashes and crash severity to the greatest extent possible. However, in many cases, practitioners have limited understanding of the potential for a treatment selection to affect road users other than those targeted by the countermeasure, or to lead to unanticipated outcomes. For instance, installing a turn lane might increase vehicle speeds or pedestrian crossing distance. A better understanding of these relationships and trade-offs should inform design choices and ultimately result in safer roadways for all users.

It is common to characterize traffic safety plans as the four "E's" of highway safety—engineering, education, enforcement, and emergency medical services. Evaluation (the fifth "E" of safety), analysis, and diagnosis of these aspects of crashes in modal and facility contexts should significantly improve the selection and design of countermeasures.

Several guides, approaches, and tools to aid the diagnostic process are already available, and the goal of this toolbox was not to reinvent the wheel, but rather to augment these existing resources. Specifically, what is lacking from the practitioner's toolbox is an integrated set of procedures, methods, and tools for conducting comprehensive diagnostic assessments of the contributing factors to crashes and for identifying matching countermeasures with a potential to improve safety performance (i.e., crash frequency and severity) and provide a meaningful return on investment to state departments of transportation (DOTs).

Specifically, existing guides and tools

- Do not provide adequate coverage of key contributing factors, such as human factors and driver behavior;
- Can be difficult to understand and hard to use and are generally not designed to be practitioner ready; and
- Do not yield actionable outcomes that include a clear description of how proposed countermeasures will increase road user safety and the design/behavioral trade-offs associated with the countermeasures.

1.2 Objectives

To address these concerns, the objectives of this project were to (1) develop new tools for diagnosing contributing factors leading to crashes that will aid practitioners in selecting appropriate countermeasures in modally diverse contexts and (2) address a wide variety of contributing factors leading to crashes (e.g., roadway, technological, behavioral, human factors, socioeconomic, demographic, weather, and land use) to further practitioner understanding of how to balance trade-off decisions.

This toolbox is not a standard and is intended to augment—not replace—the many resources that are already available on these topics. The Appendix includes brief descriptions of some existing data sources on diagnostic assessment and countermeasure selection.

1.3 How to Use This Toolbox

Intended users. The intended users of this toolbox include those involved in the planning, design, operations, or safety analyses of roadways at the federal, state, county, and city levels. This could include planners, roadway designers, traffic engineers, state safety staff, and other practitioners.

Ways to use. This toolbox is intended to provide support to those who diagnose the contributing factors that lead to crashes and to help them identify and select effective countermeasures for these crashes.

A good starting point for most users of this toolbox will be the Summary of the *Toolbox for Traffic Safety Practitioners* included as part of the front matter to this report. It is recommended to read this summary first, as it highlights the key steps and elements within the body of this toolbox, including the following:

- Safe System concepts
- The Modified Haddon Matrix
- The importance of trade-offs and evaluation activities throughout diagnostic assessment and countermeasure selection
- Human factors issues that can be included in diagnostic assessments
- The importance of selecting countermeasures that reduce the demands placed on road users, enhance their capabilities, or both

The summary also includes callouts to key chapters of the toolbox where additional information and specific tools can be found.

This toolbox can be used to assess and diagnose crashes at the national level to address broad patterns in crashes, as well as the local level to address crash clusters that could occur at specific locations. This process includes the identification and consideration of the inevitable trade-offs that must be made with respect to assessing contributing factors to crashes, especially when identifying and prioritizing countermeasures. The processes and tools provided in this toolbox also emphasize the importance of including evaluations (the fifth "E") in every stage of the diagnostic assessment/countermeasure selection process; reflecting the need to include a broad range of participants and perspectives to more fully understand why crashes occur and what can be done about them.

Chapters 2–9 of this toolbox have been developed as relatively short sections to aid rapid search and find activities on the part of the user. These chapters contain focused discussions on specific topics and include objectives, background materials, examples, and tools in the form of diagnostic questions to aid crash diagnoses, as well as flowcharts to summarize both the diagnostic assessment and countermeasure selection processes. Thus, users can obtain benefits from a mix of both (1) background knowledge that can further their understanding of key concepts and related research and concepts and (2) practical tools that identify key concepts and questions that can frame and guide the diagnostics process. Chapter 10 contains step-by-step decision trees to aid in countermeasure selection for a broad range of facility types and crash types.

1.4 Evaluation as a Key Element of Diagnostic Assessment and Countermeasure Selection

State highway safety plans (e.g., Strategic Highway Safety Plans [SHSP]) use safety data—e.g., fatal crashes and crashes involving serious injuries along with roadway and traffic data—to identify critical highway safety problems and safety improvement opportunities. These plans include specific multi-year goals, objectives, and measures to support performance-based highway programs. Specific strategies for improving safety include the highway safety elements of engineering, education, enforcement, and emergency services (the four "E's" of highway safety) (FHWA, 2016). According to FHWA (2016), "if speed is an emphasis area in a State SHSP, the State may consider a variety of 4 E strategies to reduce or mitigate the impact of speeding. Strategies might include increasing law enforcement efforts to reduce speeding (enforcement), applying traffic calming measures such as speed humps and roundabouts (engineering), delivering public information campaigns that focus on the dangers of speeding (education), and utilizing Emergency Medical Services data to quantify the burden to the health care system and the cost to the community (emergency services)."

Equally critical to improving safety performance is the evaluation (the fifth "E" of safety) of crash data in modal and facility contexts to assess and aid the selection and design of countermeasures. While program evaluation might be considered something to worry about after countermeasures have been identified, this fifth "E" should be implemented at every stage of the safety improvement process (see Figure 4) and include input and involvement from the range of transportation professionals involved, including planners, designers, engineers, and safety analysts. In short, having an evaluative mindset throughout the crash prevention process can add rigor and purpose to safety improvement planning.

Evaluation is simply the process of examining the value or worth of something. In the highway safety context, evaluations focus on rigorously analyzing and assessing the efficacy of safety

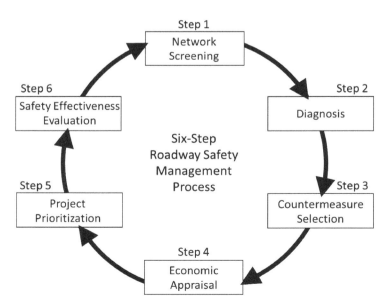

Figure 4.   Six-step safety management process (adapted from AASHTO, 2010).

improvements to determine what is working and why. As described in Pullen-Seufert and Hall (2008), evaluations should be seen as a tool to be used throughout the highway safety improvement process to clarify problems, help develop good safety questions, prioritize countermeasures, identify metrics for success, and then assess countermeasure implementations. At their most fundamental level, countermeasure evaluations focus on two basic questions: (1) did you implement the program as planned? and (2) did you accomplish your objectives? (Pullen-Seufert and Hall, 2008).

Pullen-Seufert and Hall (2008) provide a seven-step process for evaluating highway safety programs and countermeasures, as follows:

1. **Identify the problem:** Gather and analyze the information necessary to help determine the nature and size of the problem you wish to address, data on contributing factors, where the problem is manifesting, and who is being affected.
2. **Develop reasonable objectives:** What will determine the success of a proposed program, treatment, or countermeasure, and how will success be measured? Program objectives should be SMART (specific, measurable, action-oriented, reasonable, and time-specific) (Pullen-Seufert and Hall, 2008).
3. **Develop a plan for measuring results:** Develop a detailed plan that describes what you will measure, how you will measure it, and how you will analyze the results obtained. In general, evaluations are more robust when they include multiple measures obtained from multiple methods—it is beneficial to consider a range of outcome measures that are appropriate to your evaluations. For example, a countermeasure to reduce speeding behavior might use speeding-involved crashes, speeding tickets, and surveys of public awareness to assess efficacy.
4. **Gather baseline data:** Measuring the value of a proposed program, treatment, or countermeasure often includes comparing measured outcomes *before* implementation to those same outcomes *after* implementation, while controlling for other key variables that could impact the results.
5. **Implement your program:** Initiate the program, treatment, or countermeasure that is the focus of your evaluation and document all implementation issues, questions, or milestones that might be important as you analyze your data.
6. **Gather data and analyze results:** Data collection and analysis may well be the most complex and labor-intensive elements of an evaluation. In this regard, a data collection schedule with detailed procedures should be developed and followed. Pay close attention to any external events that could change your outcomes in ways that are separate from the program, treatment, or countermeasure under evaluation. For example, if you are monitoring the effects of a countermeasure to reduce speeding behavior through a specific section of roadway and that roadway undergoes a major revision involving work zones and reduced traffic and throughput, you may wish to delay the evaluation or shift the implementation to another roadway to avoid confounding the results.
7. **Report results:** Clearly communicate the objectives, methods, results, and conclusions of your evaluation to all organizations involved in the effort.

1.5 Trade-offs in a Multimodal Transportation Network

In a multimodal transportation network, trade-offs refer to the inevitable give and take around balancing multiple safety options, including assessments of the strengths and weaknesses associated with safety considerations for all road users; including drivers, pedestrians, bicyclists, and transit users. In general, trade-offs reflect a desire to achieve compromise, balance, and perhaps exchange between desirable but incompatible elements.

Thus, understanding inherent human capabilities and limitations, the broader social environment that impacts roadway safety, and how roadway infrastructure can be misaligned with them will aid practitioners in diagnosing crashes and in identifying and balancing trade-off decisions among countermeasures.

Final countermeasure selection should include trade-offs between key variables, including countermeasure efficacy, specific safety benefits, unanticipated outcomes, and feasibility (e.g., time and cost).

1.6 Summary of the Remainder of This Toolbox

This toolbox provides the safety practitioner with an integrated set of procedures, methods, and tools to support conducting diagnostic assessments of the contributing factors to crashes, identifying matching countermeasures with a potential to improve safety performance and provide a meaningful return on investment to state DOTs. Although Treat et al. (1979) found that human error was a contributing factor to over 90% of motor vehicle crashes, 27% of the crashes they investigated were caused in some part by interactions between the road infrastructure and the road user (see Table 2-1 in Treat et al., 1979). The resources for conducting comprehensive diagnostic assessments of the contributing factors to crashes described in this toolbox, therefore, focus on (1) significant contributors to crashes in terms of their influence on safety outcomes, as well as (2) topics that can be addressed by the practitioner through roadway planning, design and/or operations. The subsequent chapters in this toolbox are summarized as follows:

- **Chapter 2: What Causes Roadway Crashes?** describes key research into the causes of roadway crashes and highlights the key contributing factors that reflect interactions between driver capabilities and limitations and the demands placed on the driver by the roadway infrastructure and related traffic operations.
- **Chapter 3: Diagnostic Assessment in the Safe System** provides a holistic framework for identifying potential road-user, vehicle, environmental, social, and road-user-mix contributions to crashes and injuries issues—and their interactions—that could be impacting the safety performance of a roadway facility.
- **Chapter 4: Distinguishing Between Human Factors Issues and Aberrant Driver Behaviors** describes the differences between human factors issues and aberrant driver behaviors as contributing factors to roadway crashes and provides information that can help the practitioner distinguish between these two types of errors and mistakes.
- **Chapter 5: Perception-Response Time as a Contributing Factor to Crashes** describes the importance of the time in which drivers perceive and respond to situations ahead to avoid crashes. It discusses the various driver, environmental, and vehicle factors that can affect perception-response time, including driver expectations, visual conspicuity, and vehicle speed. Guidance is offered in how roadway elements might be designed to increase rather than decrease the perception-response time window to avoid safety-critical events.
- **Chapter 6: The Role of Expectations in Road User Behavior** discusses the importance of expectations to road user understanding of the roadway environment and provides a review of the types of expectations that road users develop and where they come from, as well as ways to assess the development of helpful versus unhelpful expectations.
- **Chapter 7: The Role of Visibility in Road User Behavior** discusses the importance of visibility on driver performance and roadway safety and how limited visibility in the driving environment can result in driver error. Diagnostic questions are included for assessing visibility concerns in roadway contexts.
- **Chapter 8: Task Demand as a Contributing Factor to Crashes** describes the importance of workload to safety and crashes. It discusses workload as the relationship between task demands and user capabilities, where task demand refers to the requirements that the facility or a maneuver within the facility places on a road user in terms of perceiving and interpreting the environment, making decisions, and then executing those decisions.

- **Chapter 9: Linking Contributing Factors to Countermeasures** emphasizes the importance of linking countermeasure identification and selection to specific human factors issues (as well as driver behavior issues) identified during the diagnostics process concerning four crash types: run-off-road, pedestrian, work zone, and intersection crashes.
- **Chapter 10: Decision Trees to Support Countermeasure Selection** shares decision trees that are provided as a visual framework to aid countermeasure selection. A series of questions are provided to help identify potential countermeasures to remedy crash patterns of interest based on crash contributing factors. Diagnostic scenarios are presented for common crash types that occur along rural and urban roadway segments and urban intersections, including pedestrian and bicycle crashes.
- **Chapter 11: Procedures for Assessing Road User Demands** provides a diagnostic method to help practitioners identify and model the key elements of the driving tasks that shape the demands placed on the road user. This chapter provides step-by-step procedures for conducting workload analysis for a given roadway segment or driving task and shows how these methods can be adapted based on the scope and resources allocated toward this effort. Examples are provided to explain how to translate the results of these analyses into recommendations for revising roadway elements and traffic operations.
- **Chapter 12: Blank Templates and Worksheets** are provided to support various data-gathering activities described within the toolbox, including key aspects of the crash diagnostics process and the process for assessing roadway workload/demand.

Figures, tables, and examples are shared throughout the text to illustrate concepts, present data, and provide templates for practitioner use. Some of these materials appear in more than one chapter to facilitate usage of the varied tools. The chapters of the report are followed by the references, a list of acronyms and abbreviations, and the Appendix.

CHAPTER 2

What Causes Roadway Crashes?

2.1 Objectives

The objectives of this tool are to

- Summarize research into the contributing factors to roadway crashes,
- Present basic human factors concepts and describe how they relate to driving, and
- Describe the four key human factors contributors to crashes.

2.2 Background

Successful safety management practices—including the selection of properly focused and cost-effective countermeasures—depend on an accurate understanding of the underlying contributing causes of crashes. To aid both diagnostics and design activities, researchers have been exploring ways to approach and model accidents (including roadway crashes) for many years (for a useful summary, see Coury et al., 2010).

Summary of research into crash causality. Building on this earlier work that focused on industrial accidents, plane crashes, railroad derailments, and nuclear power incidents, more recent research studies and governmental investigations have applied these general approaches to roadway crash causation, in which they fostered ideas about how to prevent crashes from occurring and about implementing countermeasures. For example, in 1979, Treat and colleagues published a seminal report for the United States Department of Transportation (U.S. DOT) that showed in an analysis of over 2,000 motor vehicle crashes that nearly 93% were caused in some part by human factors; more specifically, they identified improper lookout, excessive speed, and inattention as the top reasons for crashes because of human factors issues (Treat et al., 1979). Figure 5 summarizes the results.

Other probable causes for crashes included environmental factors such as view obstructions and slick roads, as well as vehicular factors such as brake failure and tire underinflation. Treat et al. (1979) suggested several countermeasures that are still relevant today, substantiating the notion that most of these crashes are indeed caused by human factors-related issues rather than vehicular or environmental factors that would otherwise be solved with advances in automotive technology or improved infrastructure.

In 2008, the National Highway Traffic Safety Administration (NHTSA) conducted the National Motor Vehicle Crash Causation Survey (NMVCCS), in which 6,950 crashes from 2005 to 2007 were evaluated (NHTSA, 2008a; Singh, 2015). The results acquired from this survey allowed for identifying common pre-crash events and scenarios, such as turning or crossing at intersections, and for determining critical reasons underlying these events, which include driver errors, vehicle and environmental conditions, and roadway design. The National Transportation

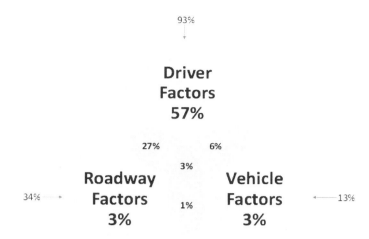

Figure 5. Relative roles of driver, environmental, and vehicle factors in crashes (adapted from Treat et al., 1979).

Safety Board (NTSB) has also helped clarify the contributing factors of crashes by generating detailed investigative reports of numerous transportation crashes, which identify major safety issues and assess the efficacy of traffic control measures in protecting pedestrians and vehicles from crashes (NTSB, 2004; NTSB, 2009). These investigative reports have resulted in recommendations for improving roadway safety and preventing crashes.

Most recently, Dong and Wood (2023) assessed the contributing factors to crashes using 2017–2020 data from the Crash Investigation Sampling System (CISS) (NHTSA, n.d.b) and 2010–2015 data from the National Automotive Sampling System (NASS) Crashworthiness Data System (NHTSA, n.d.d) using taxonomies that included those used by Treat et al. (1979) and Singh (2015) (i.e., human factors, vehicle factors, and roadway and environmental factors). These data sets are very detailed and include police-reported crash information, crash reconstructions, hospital data, and interviews of people involved in the collisions. The findings were overall very similar to those reported previously; more than 95% of the crashes investigated involved human factors or included a human error.

Nature and types of driver errors. The concept that humans play a fundamental role in roadway crashes has been utilized to develop taxonomies to better understand and assess the driver errors that lead to crashes. To elaborate, in the 1990s, James Reason detailed how the psychological nature of humans contributes to accident causation by categorizing the types of errors that they commit into two groups: (1) slips (i.e., unplanned actions), lapses (i.e., covert memory failures) and mistakes (i.e., planning or problem-solving failures); and (2) violations (i.e., motivational problems) (Reason, 1995). Reason began developing such distinctions between categories by having individuals complete a driver behavior questionnaire, which asked them to judge the frequency with which they committed various types of errors and violations when driving (Reason et al., 1990). From these results, Reason identified three factors: violations, dangerous errors, and relatively harmless lapses. These survey results emphasized the view that different psychological mechanisms mediate errors and violations when driving. For example, individuals who reported having the most violations tended to rate themselves as skillful drivers, errors and lapses when driving involved cognitive competence (e.g., attentional) failures, and violations involved the motivational factors of the driver (Reason et al., 1990). Taken together, these findings highlight the importance of considering the driver's psychological state when assessing the errors and violations involved in crash causation.

Driver error categorization has been used as a methodology by others to create more specific categories in the formation of diagnostic tools, such as checklists and questionnaires, that may be used for assessing the causes of roadway crashes. Wierwille et al. (2002) collected data from focus groups with police officers and interviews with drivers involved in crashes to develop a novel taxonomy to describe driver errors, which included topics such as inadequate knowledge, training, and skill; impairment; willful inappropriate behavior; and infrastructure or environment problems (Wierwille et al., 2002). These topics highlighted the need to consider not only willful violations but also how drivers interact with the surrounding infrastructure features; this concept is exemplified by organizing the driver-related issues into a tree diagram that branches off into other contributing psychology- and infrastructure-related components (Wierwille et al., 2002). For example, failure to yield at an intersection may be the general category that describes the crash type, but that kind of driver error may branch off into more particular components, like the type of intersection (infrastructure-related) and specific reasons for not yielding (related to human factors) (Wierwille et al., 2002).

Most crashes reflect multiple contributing causal factors. Crashes are complex, and multiple converging elements are associated with many roadway crashes. Thus, an effective framework and methodology for the diagnostic assessment of crashes should include not just a review and analysis of relevant road user, environmental, and vehicle factors but also the interactions between these factors. This perspective is emphasized by the crash trifecta concept, which includes unsafe pre-incident behavior or maneuvers; transient driver inattention; and unexpected traffic events. The first element of the crash trifecta, unsafe pre-incident behavior or maneuvers, includes actions that are typically under the driver's control and may occur before the safety-critical event. Examples of this element include speeding, tailgating, and making an unsafe turn (Dunn et al., 2014). The second element is transient driver inattention, which may or may not be related to the act of driving. For instance, a driver may be suddenly distracted when checking mirrors to determine whether or not they could safely move to the adjacent lane.

However, the driver may also become transiently distracted if their mobile phone falls on the car floor and they reach to retrieve it, which is not linked to the act of driving itself (Dunn et al., 2014). The final element of the crash trifecta includes an unexpected traffic event, which refers to an unexpected action or random event committed by another vehicle or obstacle, such as a deer suddenly running out in front of the vehicle (Dunn et al., 2014). Taken together, these three elements make clear that factors contributing to many vehicle crashes involve an interaction between driver-related and non-driver-related factors and events.

Looking at the role of interactions between contributing factors is not a new perspective on crashes; the Haddon Matrix (Haddon, 1972; Haddon, 1980) has long provided a technique and tool for looking at factors related to personal attributes, vehicle attributes, and environmental attributes before, during, and after an injury or death. Human factors evaluations of crashes have similar goals: to conduct site-specific human factors evaluations and to consider and list the individual road user, vehicle, and environment factors (plus interactions) that could contribute to driver confusion, misperceptions, high workload, or other mistakes and errors. In this regard, Campbell et al. (2018) proposed using the Human Factors Interaction Matrix (HFIM) to specifically identify road users and other factors that could contribute to driver errors across a range of various scenarios and driving situations.

Critically then, it is often the interactions among road users, vehicles, and the environment that lead to errors, conflicts, crashes, and fatalities. Errors made by road users do not generally reflect the breakdown or occurrence of a single factor; they reflect a confluence of factors that occur more or less simultaneously. For example, a crash does not generally happen just because a driver is older; rather, it might happen to an older driver driving at night, under bad weather conditions, when faced with a sign that may be wordy, complicated, damaged, or worn out. This emphasis on the role of interactions in crashes is well-supported by crash-data research such as that reported by Treat et al. (1979) and Singh (2015).

2.3 Key Concepts: Contributing Factors to Roadway Crashes

Human factors refer to the role of user capabilities and limitations in crashes. As shown in Figure 5, while most crashes reflect some sort of driver error, some of these errors (approximately 57%) reflect driver behavior issues, such as impaired driving because of drugs or alcohol, road rage, fatigue, and distraction/inattention, while others (approximately 30%) reflect human factors issues, that is, roadway designs and traffic operation features that unknowingly place demands on road users that may exceed their capabilities. Chapter 3 describes the distinctions between these types of contributing factors and provides some diagnostic questions that will aid the practitioner in discerning between them. The chapter briefly introduces human factors and identifies the key ways in which roadway designs and traffic operation features can place demands on road users that may exceed their capabilities.

The study of human factors applies knowledge from human sciences such as psychology, physiology, sociology, and kinesiology to the design of systems, tasks, and environments to promote and support safe and effective use. The goal of understanding the effects of human factors is to reduce the probability and consequences of human error—especially the injuries and fatalities resulting from these errors—by designing systems, tasks, and environments that consider inherent, relatively stable human capabilities and limitations.

These human capabilities and limitations are relevant to roadway design, driver performance, and the general safety performance of a roadway. The roadway system reflects complex interactions between different road users (e.g., drivers, pedestrians, and bicyclists), vehicle types (e.g., cars, motorcycles, trucks, and trains), and elements in the environment (e.g., roadways, markings, signs, and weather conditions). The design of the roadway system impacts numerous safety-relevant behaviors on the part of drivers, such as where they are looking as they drive, how they maintain their lane position, and how they select their speed. These behaviors have been studied by human factors researchers and practitioners for many years. Drivers make frequent mistakes because of their physical, perceptual, and cognitive limitations; some of these mistakes may lead to conflicts between road users or even near misses, but others may lead to crashes that result in injuries or deaths.

What are these capabilities and limitations, and how do they relate to driving, a pedestrian trying to cross a street, or a bicyclist sharing the roadway with vehicles? Capabilities and limitations may be summarized by reference to a human information processing model, which is a frequent and convenient way to represent how humans relate to their environment (Wickens, 1992). In a nutshell, as a road user directs their attention to the environment, their senses receive and process raw information (i.e., they see, hear, and feel); they interpret and organize this information into more concrete perceptions; they store that information in memory and then use that information (along with other information they have stored in the past) to make decisions and execute responses.

While a thorough review of the human information processing model is beyond the scope of this chapter, suffice it to say that these processes—seeing, perceiving, remembering, deciding, and responding—have elements and constraints that reflect the inherent physical and mental abilities of all road users. For example,

- Seeing requires having sufficient light and visual contrast between an object and its background;
- Perceiving involves an awareness of the elements within the environment, such as the speed and distance of approaching vehicles;

- Remembering includes memory of traffic rules or of the meanings of signs passed;
- Deciding involves knowledge, mental ability; and
- Responding requires physical ability and time.

These information-processing elements translate into roadway design principles that will support accurate and timely behaviors from drivers and other road users. While there are differences in these capabilities and limitations across individuals (e.g., older versus younger drivers), proficiency (e.g., experienced versus inexperienced drivers), and circumstances (distracted versus unimpaired driving), they vary within relatively restricted and well-known boundaries. For example, vision is the primary source for obtaining information while operating a motor vehicle, and researchers have estimated that as much as 90% of the information needed for the driving task is obtained through vision, highlighting the importance of treating roadways as an information system (Dewar and Olson, 2007). Roadways are always sending messages to the road user. The roadway designer should aim to design the road in such a way that the right messages are being sent at the right time.

Driving example: responding to an advance warning sign. Consider the information processing elements and the roadway as an information system in the context of a simple and common driving activity such as slowing a car in response to a sharp curve in the road. See the example in the text box.

> Suppose a driver is approaching a curve in the roadway and sees a roadway sign just ahead of the curve that provides an advance warning ("Curve Ahead" sign) of the approaching curve. The driver sees the sign, processes the words on the sign (including other cues such as sign color, shape, and location), and then recognizes the sign given the driving context. The driver processes the curve itself as well and, based on features such as lane width, radius, and current speed, re-assesses the current vehicle speed. From the driver's perception of current speed and memory about the sign's meaning given the driving context, the driver determines that the sign means it is necessary to slow down. The driver decides to slow down, and then lets off on the accelerator and steps on the brake in such a way as to slow down at the right location to support positioning within the curve that is efficient and keeps the vehicle within the lane boundaries.

Table 4 integrates the description of human information processing elements with this simple task of slowing a car in response to a sharp curve in the road; consider how different roadway elements combine to communicate with and provide messages to the driver. In the table, the sensation, perception, and attention elements might be characterized as the active information-seeking portions of driving; the decision-making element is where the driver determines what to do; and the response execution element includes the physical acts involved in making steering, accelerator, and brake inputs to the vehicle. However, the elements do not necessarily occur in a fixed sequence, and under most circumstances, they reflect a series of stages with multiple feedback loops and no fixed starting point.

Human factors are important to highway safety because human factors issues related to the infrastructure can contribute to driver errors, and such errors can—in turn—contribute to crashes. Many crashes occur when the demands of the roadway environment exceed the capabilities of the roadway user. For example, the roadway can include objects that you cannot see because of limitations in your visual abilities (e.g., a dark-clad pedestrian at night), or it can require you

Table 4.   Application of the information processing model of human capabilities to a simple driving task.

Human Information Processing Element	Description	Application of the Curve Ahead Sign to What the Driver Does
Attention	Actively processing information—can occur unconsciously or under active control	Focusing awareness on the critical aspects of the roadway environment
Sensation	Seeing, hearing, feeling	Sensing specific features of the environment—the roadway, lane width and edges, and the Curve Ahead sign
Perception	Organizing and interpreting senses into a coherent "picture" through a series of top-down (context, whole scene) and bottom-up (individual elements) processes	Extracting meaning from the scene by using aspects of the environment such as color and luminance gradients, separations between the roadway itself and scene elements on the roadway, and the relative location of these scene elements
Decision-making	Selecting between response options	What to do? Deciding to slow down and to adjust steering
Response Execution	Acting, doing	Releasing the accelerator, pressing the brake in a controlled manner, and matching steering inputs to road curvature
Memory	Retaining and recalling	Supporting the entire task by providing meaning to the sign, based on knowledge and past experience with this stretch of roadway

to respond to changing conditions faster than you can perceive and respond to these conditions (e.g., an off-ramp that is too close to a decision point).

Even crashes associated with impaired driving fit this "demands versus capabilities" framework, as impaired driving (e.g., driving while drunk or under the influence of drugs, distracted driving, fatigued driving) can reduce baseline capabilities related to information processing elements such as vision, perception, decision-making, and response times. For example, distracted driving may reduce the time available to perceive and extract important information from the roadway environment, drugs may impair decision-making abilities, and alcohol may slow response times to roadway hazards. Thus, understanding inherent human capabilities and limitations and how roadway infrastructure can be misaligned with them will aid practitioners in diagnosing crashes and in identifying and balancing trade-off decisions among countermeasures.

2.3.1 Human Factors and the Demands of the Driving Task

While the tools for diagnostic assessment summarized in Chapter 1 include behavioral elements (i.e., road users' responses to the roadway environment), they can lack insights to help clarify the relationships between roadway design and operations decisions, crash frequency and severity outcomes, and the underlying needs and characteristics of road users. In keeping with the role that user errors and mistakes play in roadway crashes (Treat et al., 1979; Wierwille et al., 2002; Singh, 2015), the tools provided in this toolbox incorporate and refer to human factors topics (i.e., interactions between the road user and the infrastructure) and address roadway design from an engineering standpoint.

When task demands exceed user capabilities, crashes are more likely. The discussions in several sections of this chapter focus on the important role that demands play in road user performance and—in general—the safety performance of a roadway. Indeed, understanding how drivers interact with the roadway allows highway agencies to plan and construct highways in a manner that minimizes human error and its resultant crashes. A key premise of this toolbox is that human factors are important to highway safety because human factors issues related to the infrastructure can contribute to driver errors, and such errors contribute to crashes. In short, many crashes happen when the demands of the roadway environment exceed the capabilities of the roadway user.

Driving involves a complex series of physical actions and mental operations that vary considerably across driving contexts, situations, and conditions. For example, there are differences in the demands and effort associated with merging onto a busy urban freeway at night compared to driving a long section of freeway with light traffic in the middle of the day. Another approach is to link specific features of the driving environment with the information processing elements through a more detailed task analysis of driver activities and associated demands. Task analysis is a technique that can be used to describe any goal-oriented set of human activities. It typically includes the successive decomposition of a high-level activity into smaller elements (e.g., segments, tasks, and subtasks) with specific information processing elements and workload estimates developed at the subtask level. The technique is highly flexible in terms of how information may be generated (e.g., through observations, interviews, or expert analysis) and how task details are presented (e.g., from the simple text presented in tabular form to complex graphical depictions).

The driver demands associated with navigating a curve were illustrated in a task analysis included in the *Human Factors Guidelines for Road Systems* (HFG) (Campbell et al., 2012) and can serve as an example of how analyzing driver tasks can be helpful for understanding how roadway design impacts driver performance. Figure 6 describes the activities that drivers would typically perform while navigating a single horizontal curve. From this example, it is evident that certain tasks—like maintaining speed and lane position while entering and following the curve—are more demanding and challenge the driver to pay closer attention to basic vehicle control and visual information acquisition. Also, since the task analysis identifies the key information and vehicle control elements in different parts of the curve driving task, Figure 6 illustrates how and when driver demands are influenced by design aspects such as design consistency, degree of curvature, and lane width. In particular, identifying highly demanding (or high-workload) components of the curve driving task indicates where drivers might benefit from information regarding delineation or benefit from the elimination of potential visual distractions. The concept of driver demands and workload is discussed in more detail in Chapters 8 and 11.

2.3.2 Key Human Factors Issues Associated with Crashes

Human factors issues as contributors to roadway crashes have been the subject of empirical studies for decades, with many such studies summarized in the HFG (Campbell et al., 2012). These studies have identified several human factors issues that are frequently linked to crashes. For example, the recent *Primer on the Joint Use of the Highway Safety Manual (HSM) and the Human Factors Guidelines (HFG) for Road Systems* (Campbell et al., 2018) identified several candidate human factors issues, including age, visual capabilities, driving experience, cognitive ability, language/culture, road familiarity, physical abilities, attitudes, and training (in addition to driver behavior issues). Though this set of candidate issues provides a good foundation for understanding of the role of human factors issues in crashes, it is too broad and lengthy to serve as the core of a crash diagnostics process. In general, it is important to focus on those human factors issues that reflect (1) significant contributors to crashes in terms of their influence on

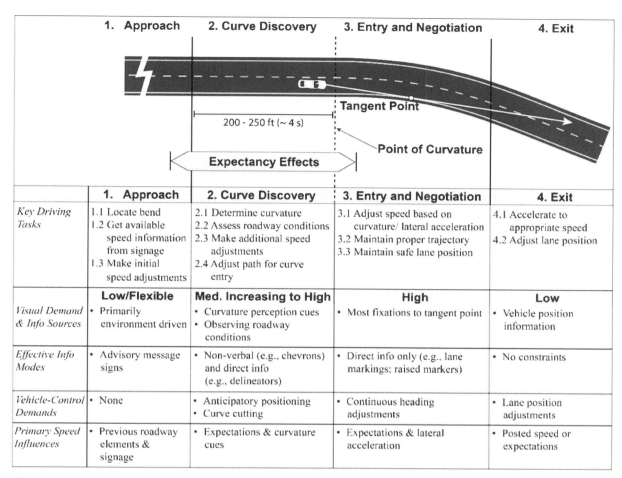

	1. Approach	**2. Curve Discovery**	**3. Entry and Negotiation**	**4. Exit**
Key Driving Tasks	1.1 Locate bend 1.2 Get available speed information from signage 1.3 Make initial speed adjustments	2.1 Determine curvature 2.2 Assess roadway conditions 2.3 Make additional speed adjustments 2.4 Adjust path for curve entry	3.1 Adjust speed based on curvature/ lateral acceleration 3.2 Maintain proper trajectory 3.3 Maintain safe lane position	4.1 Accelerate to appropriate speed 4.2 Adjust lane position
Visual Demand & Info Sources	**Low/Flexible** • Primarily environment driven	**Med. Increasing to High** • Curvature perception cues • Observing roadway conditions	**High** • Most fixations to tangent point	**Low** • Vehicle position information
Effective Info Modes	• Advisory message signs	• Non-verbal (e.g., chevrons) and direct info (e.g., delineators)	• Direct info only (e.g., lane markings; raised markers)	• No constraints
Vehicle-Control Demands	• None	• Anticipatory positioning • Curve cutting	• Continuous heading adjustments	• Lane position adjustments
Primary Speed Influences	• Previous roadway elements & signage	• Expectations & curvature cues	• Expectations & lateral acceleration	• Posted speed or expectations

Figure 6.   Example of driver demands when navigating a horizontal curve (adapted from Campbell et al., 2012).

safety performance and (2) topics that can be addressed by the practitioner through roadway planning, design, and/or operations.

In this regard, several relevant human factors data sources [e.g., Wierwille et al., 2002; Campbell et al., 2012; Theeuwes and van der Horst, 2012; Theeuwes, 2021; Permanent International Association of Road Congresses (PIARC), 2016; PIARC, 2019a] make clear that four human factors topics in particular are key to the efficacy of roadways as information systems and the general safety performance of roadways: perception-response time, expectations, visibility, and workload. This toolbox provides more detailed descriptions and diagnostic questions associated with each of these key human factors-related contributors to crashes. The following summarizes each factor:

- **Perception-Response Time:** The facility should provide enough time for road users to perceive, then decide, and then respond/act.
- **Expectations:** The facility should be laid out logically, be consistent with road user expectations, and avoid confusing users.
- **Visibility:** The facility should support the visual perception and comprehension of relevant objects in the environment.
- **Workload:** The facility should not place demands on road users that are inconsistent with their inherent capabilities (e.g., perceptual/visual, decision-making, and physical capabilities).

As important as these contributing factors are to crashes, these factors should not be considered in isolation from one another or from other factors that might contribute to crashes. As noted earlier, errors made by road users do not generally reflect the breakdown or occurrence of a single factor; they reflect a confluence of factors that occur more or less simultaneously. Specifically, it is often the interactions among road users, vehicles, and the environment that lead to errors, conflicts, crashes, and fatalities (Dingus et al., 2006). As noted recently by Hauer (2020), crashes usually have more than one cause, and "[a] crash cause is a circumstance or action that, were it different, the frequency of crashes and/or their severity would be different" (p. 4). Thus, an effective framework and methodology for the diagnostic assessment of crashes must include not just a review and analysis of relevant road user, environmental, and vehicle factors, but also the interactions between these factors (see also the HFIM from Campbell et al., 2018). For example, a crash does not generally happen just because a driver is older; rather, it might happen to an older driver driving at night, under bad weather conditions, when faced with a sign that may be wordy, complicated, damaged, or worn out.

PIARC Human Factors Guidelines highlights "three classes of human factors accident triggers in the man-road interface":

1. The road should give the driver enough time to react safely (time).
2. The road must offer a safe field of view (visibility).
3. The road has to follow the driver's perception logic (expectations) (PIARC, 2016, p. 13).

The HFG (Campbell et al., 2012) is closely aligned with these highlights in the PIARC document, with numerous guidelines addressing the importance of time, visibility, and expectations. The HFG—consistent with general guidance for all person-machine interactions—also focuses on the crucial topic of demand or workload. Indeed, the crash record makes it clear that the overwhelming majority of crashes in which driver error plays a role involve situations in which the demands of the driving task exceed the driver's capabilities (Treat et al., 1979; Singh, 2015). Thus, to time, visibility, and expectations, workload is added to those human factors topics that reflect key contributors to crashes.

Key Concepts

1. While the great majority of crashes involve some type of driver error, it is often the interactions among road users, vehicles, and the environment that lead to crashes.
2. Many crashes occur when the demands of the roadway environment exceed the capabilities of the roadway user.
3. Roadways are always sending messages to the road user—the key is to design the road so that the right messages are provided at the right time.
4. Four human factors issues are key to the safety performance of roadways: (1) perception-response time, (2) driver expectations, (3) visibility, and (4) workload/demand.

2.4 Diagnostic Questions Related to the Contributing Factors to Roadway Crashes

As a designer or traffic engineer, consider if and how your roadway places demands on users that might be greater than their inherent capabilities:

- Consider the individual roadway elements (e.g., signs, markings, traffic lights, lane widths, shoulder widths) present within the facility under study:
  - What messages are these individual elements likely to be communicating to the typical road user?
    - Is this the message you intend to communicate?
      - If not, consider how to communicate your message more effectively.
    - Is the message being communicated in the right way?
      - If not, consider alternative methods for communicating to road users [e.g., adding signs to augment lane markings, adding dynamic roadway features, or Transportation Systems Management and Operations (TSM&O) strategies to support timely communications to road users (AASHTO, n.d.b)].
    - Is the message being communicated at the right time and place?
      - If not, consider relocating signs or other elements to a location where they will be more effective.
- Consider both the individual roadway elements (e.g., signs, markings, traffic lights, lane widths, shoulder widths) and the broader facility under study:
  - Does it seem that road users may have insufficient time to respond to typical demands?
    - If yes, see Chapter 5: "Perception-Response Time as a Contributing Factor to Crashes" for more information.
  - Does it seem that some roadway features may be inconsistent with what users might expect or include abrupt changes in driving requirements?
    - If yes, see Chapter 6: "The Role of Expectations in Road User Behavior" for more information.
  - Does it seem that road users may have problems seeing or perceiving key roadway elements under a range of operating conditions (e.g., day and night)?
    - If yes, see Chapter 7: "The Role of Visibility in Road User Behavior" for more information.
  - Does it seem that some typical or required tasks associated with the roadway may place excessive demands on the capabilities of a typical user?
    - If yes, see Chapter 8: "Task Demand as a Contributing Factor to Crashes" for more information.

CHAPTER 3

Diagnostic Assessment in the Safe System

3.1 Objectives

The objectives of this tool are to provide the following:

- A Safe System approach to help identify potential contributions to crashes and injuries that could be impacting the safety performance of a roadway.
- A process for assessing crash and site data to summarize patterns and findings related to contributing factors.
- Diagnostic questions to help identify crash patterns, crash types, and contributing factors.

3.2 Background

Traditional models of crash causation that take into account potential hazards at various stages may not sufficiently consider the complex and often nuanced relationships between all road users and roadway features. For example, assigning a single, unitary crash-relevant conflict as the proximal cause of a safety-critical event without considering additional contributing factors is a limitation and would not address all the factors involved in the cause of crashes (Dunn et al., 2014). This emphasis on the role of interactions in roadway crashes is well-supported by crash data (Treat et al., 1979). Figure 5 in Chapter 2 shows that while drivers contributed to 93% of crashes, they were the sole cause of only 57% of crashes; the crash percentages in the shaded regions of the figure highlight the role of driver/roadway/vehicle interactions as causal factors in crashes. Similarly, traditional approaches may not address the needs of all road users (e.g., bicyclists and pedestrians) or the pre- and post-crash factors that might influence injury prevention and reduction.

The Safe System approach seeks to create a road environment that maximizes safety performance by not accepting that death and serious injury are a natural consequence of using a road system (Finkel et al., 2020; Signor et al., 2018; Welle et al., 2018). Rather than relying primarily on improving human behavior, this approach seeks to plan, design, and operate a road system that recognizes humans make mistakes, have limited physiological abilities to safely negotiate complex situations, and have a limited tolerance of kinetic energy forces. The Safe System approach incorporates five elements: safe road users, safe vehicles, safe speeds, safe roads, and post-crash care. The fifth "E" (evaluation) should exist at every stage of the safety management process and not just toward the end of the process as part of countermeasure evaluation, meaning that the diagnostic process should be considered an evaluative activity.

A goal of this approach is to create a system that reduces the risk of kinetic energy transfer occurring in the first place and reduces the amount of energy transfer in the event of a crash to an amount that can be tolerated by humans. Part B of the HSM (AASHTO, 2010) provides methods for network screening and crash diagnosis to understand potential contributing factors and identify treatments and methods for selecting and prioritizing projects. The HSM does support an approach to crash diagnostics that would reveal multiple contributing factors. However, it provides few procedures for assessing a broad range of driver/roadway interactions and does not incorporate the holistic approach envisioned by Safe System. The systems approach advocated by Safe System applies not just to planning and design activities, but also to the procedures for diagnosing crashes and identifying focused countermeasures to address them. In short, holistic design and countermeasure selection require a holistic approach to crash diagnostics.

3.3 Key Concepts: A Safe System Approach to Diagnostic Assessment

William Haddon developed the Haddon Matrix to improve emergency responses for people injured in crashes and provide a technique and tool for looking at factors related to personal attributes, vehicle attributes, and environmental attributes before, during, and after an injury or death (Haddon, 1972; Haddon, 1980). The goal of applying this type of tool is to help the practitioner think about and list the individual road user, vehicle, and environment factors (and any possible interactions) that could contribute to driver confusion, misperceptions, high workload, distraction, or other problems and errors. Research studies and governmental investigations have applied the Haddon Matrix to roadway crash causation to generate ideas on crash prevention and countermeasure implementation.

Haddon's epidemiological view of injury outlines three phases: (1) A pre-crash phase with those factors that influence whether a crash will occur and result in injuries; (2) A crash event phase with those factors that influence injury severity during the crash event; and (3) a post-crash phase with those factors that influence the survivability of the crash after the event (for a summary, see also: Haddon, 1972; National Committee for Injury Prevention and Control, 1989). Haddon's original matrix included examining contributory factors to these phases according to human, vehicle, environmental, and socioeconomic factors. To augment this approach, Milton and van Schalkwyk (J. Milton and I. van Schalkwyk, personal communication, January 17, 2022) have developed a framework that considers all road users (e.g., the volume of biking and walking) and the supporting social safety environment. Consistent with the Safe System approach, it includes user-mix considerations and interactions between these factors (see also the HFIM in Campbell et al., 2018). Table 5 shows a Modified Haddon Matrix (developed by John Milton and Ida van Schalkwyk of the Washington State Department of Transportation and used with their kind permission) applied to crashes in the Safe System.

This modification of the original Haddon and Human Factor Interaction Matrices aims to present a framework that more directly considers all road users and the supporting social safety environment. In doing so, these characteristics are highlighted to provide safety professionals an expanded view of the issues related to human factors within the Safe System approach.

By introducing social environment factors, safety professionals are asked to consider the implications of attitudes, biases, and equity decision-making frameworks for humans operating in the roadway environment. Doing so expands the potential diagnostic assessments that safety professionals perform. It considers laws intended to reduce potential severity (Signor et al., 2018) or the frequency of crashes and the road user's willingness to accept those laws to process the importance of understanding their current situation (e.g., high level of speeding, drinking/drugs, mid-block crossings) and how these can be used to address potential safety outcomes. Furthermore, equity is considered since it may not be correct to assume accessibility to vehicles or to personal protective equipment (PPE), especially within a particular location (e.g., a lower-income and overburdened community) where road users may not have the income to purchase a vehicle or a bicycle helmet. Moreover, in their respective community, sidewalks and pedestrian lighting may not exist, leading to lower levels of safety and security.

Table 5. Modified Haddon Matrix applied to motor vehicle crashes in the Safe System.

Phases	Human	Vehicle	Physical Environment/ Context	Social Environment	User-Mix Considerations	Interactions Between Users
Pre-event (*Before the crash occurs*) **Factors that may increase the likelihood of the crash before the crash event**	• Driver's perceptual, cognitive, and physical abilities • Alcohol and drug impairment • Impairment from fatigue • Distraction • Driver experience • Ability to perceive and react to unexpected events in a driving environment (e.g., understanding the potential for different road users) • Alertness/attentiveness • Familiarity with route • Expectations for the environment/facility	• Maintenance of brakes, tires • Speed of travel • Load characteristics • Size of vehicle • Safety and/or driver assistance features • Type of vehicle (e.g., commercial vehicle, passenger vehicle, motorcycle, bicycle, scooter)	• Roadway markings • Divided highways • Roadway lighting • Intersection type and angle • Road curvature • Signage • Walking and biking availability, facility type, separation • Roadway shoulders • Ambient and vehicle lighting	• Public attitudes on drinking and driving • Impaired driving laws • Graduated licensing laws • Seat belt, helmet, and other personal protective equipment laws • Risky behavior prominence • Support for injury prevention efforts • Positive Safety Culture • Equity considerations for lower income (e.g, PPE, Driver Ed., scholarships) • Presence of passengers	• Volume of walking and biking • Type and separation of path/shoulder sidewalk • Route directness • Crossing distance from generators • Reliance on transit, walking, and biking • Lighting Scale • Sense of security of routes • Intersection turning speeds and priorities for operations • Mid-Block Crossing controls • Intersection type • Speed management	• Speed setting consistent with user mix • Ability to maintain consistent operating speeds • Choice-making based on road users' safety and security • Common Behaviors • Education and enforcement • Ability to turn on red, permitted, and protected signals for vulnerable road users (VRUs) • Access management
Event (*During the crash*) **Factors that may influence the injury or severity of the crash during the crash event**	• Spread out energy in time and space with seat belt and/or airbag use • Child restraint use • Personal protective gear	• Vehicle size (also consider mass and center of gravity) • Crashworthiness of vehicle, overall safety rating • Airbags (type and placement) • Padded dashboards and steering wheel	• Guard rails, median barriers, breakaway devices • Presence of fixed objects near the roadway • Roadside embankments • Other road users	• Seat belt, child restraint, and other PPE laws are followed • Enforcement of occupant restraint laws • Motorcycle and bicycle helmet laws or use or both are followed and accepted	• Travel speeds • Vehicle size and type • Design exposure that tends to increase speed or threats during crossing or walking on facilities • Separation of users • Proximity of VRUs to vehicles	• Speeds resulting in injury • Angle of crash through design and operation • Vision, speed judgment • Protective equipment and restraint use • Crash-worthy roadside hardware and clear zone
Post-event (*After the crash*) **Factors that may influence the survivability of the crash after the event**	• Crash victim's general health status • Age of victims	• Gas tanks designed to maintain integrity during a crash to minimize fires • Ability to extract injured • Vehicle size, mass, and center of gravity	• Availability of effective EMS systems • Ability to respond quickly to crash • Distance to trauma care • Rehabilitation programs in place	• Public support for an emergency, trauma care, and post-crash rehabilitation • EMS training	• Trauma center availability and proximity • Emergency response	• Redundancy of system • Ability to respond and transport to care

Note: A blank template of this matrix is available in Chapter 12.

Most often, road-user mix is not an explicit consideration in safety decision-making. The Modified Haddon Matrix is intended to help practitioners assess all road users' perspectives—not just those of vehicle drivers—and to consider how decisions are made by those walking, biking, or rolling on the road. It is also intended for the safety professional to consider potential human factors related to the relationship between vehicle drivers and VRUs (e.g., difficulties associated with judging closing speed and distance or that a VRU may not be recognized, seen, or reacted to).

3.4 A General Tool and Process for Diagnostic Assessment

A diagnostic assessment process that incorporates holistic elements is not markedly different from the diagnosis procedures traditionally used by practitioners and documented in sources like the HSM (AASHTO, 2010) and the HSM/HFG *Primer* (Campbell et al., 2018). It explicitly incorporates not just general consideration of road users but also

- Considers pre-, during-, and post-crash factors that might have contributed to the crash itself, as well as post-crash survivability;
- Addresses specific issues related to the role of expectations, visibility, workload, and perception-response time in crashes; and
- Produces a detailed summary of possible contributing factors as well as their likely interactions.

The discussion in this section and the steps depicted in Figure 7 are adapted from *Primer on the Joint Use of the Highway Safety Manual (HSM) and the Human Factors Guidelines (HFG) for Road Systems* (Campbell et al., 2018) that was developed to provide the practitioner with information from both the HSM and the HFG to aid in assessing the contributing factors to crashes and selecting countermeasures.

In addressing the information in the Modified Haddon Matrix (Table 5), the objective is to consider and document the possible road user, vehicle, and environment issues that could contribute to confusion, errors, and crashes at the site or traffic situation that is under evaluation. While addressing a broader range of pre-, during-, and post-crash factors is desirable and supportive

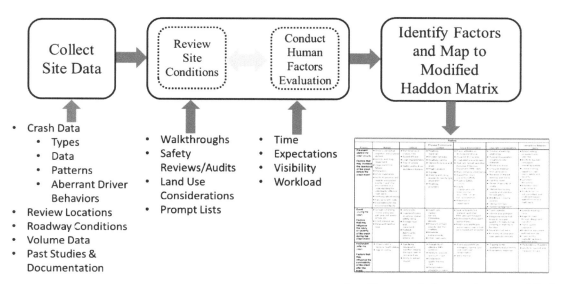

Consider pre-, during-, and post-crash factors

Figure 7.   A general process for diagnostic assessment in the Safe System.

of Safe System, valuable information supporting possible countermeasures can be obtained through a more modest analysis of the crash, site, and human factors data. Key inputs to the development process of a Modified Haddon Matrix include

- The basic crash or conflict data compiled in the site visit results (including relevant site data, such as the types of vehicles, cross-section dimensions, traffic volumes, speed limits, and the kind of traffic control),
- Considerations of infrastructure elements upstream of individual crash sites, and
- The crash data summaries.

At this early stage, it is best to generate a Modified Haddon Matrix that includes all possible factors impacting safety performance. Specifically, the matrix should include any factors and combinations of factors (interactions) that could reasonably contribute to the known or suspected opportunities for reducing crash potentials at the site under investigation. Broad considerations should include crash or conflict type, frequency, severity, and contributing factors, as well as on-the-scene observations of the facility and representative traffic movements (including pedestrians, bicyclists, and transit vehicles). In this regard, some interactions may be quantitative and very specific, while others may be qualitative and reflect possible impacts.

The diagnostic process can consider both context classification and functional classification during the identification of contributing factors to crashes. In particular, consideration of the position and type of service being provided by roadways (traditional functional classification), the environment surrounding the roadway, and how the roadway fits into and serves the community and multimodal needs and issues (context classification) can be helpful to crash diagnostics.

Most crashes (or conflicts and near-misses) will result from interactions among two or more of the individual factors. Therefore, identifying known or possible crash- or conflict-relevant interactions will be critical for identifying possible countermeasures. As a virtual road user, carefully think through ways in which the individual factors could—in combination—create confusion, distraction, uncertainties, or misperceptions on the part of actual road users. Document those factors likely to negatively affect driving scenarios and road user behaviors, especially considering the site-specific crash and safety data.

This chapter's discussion regarding a process for diagnostic assessment is intended to support populating the Modified Haddon Matrix to the extent possible. Figure 7 summarizes this part of the process and is primarily intended to emphasize the importance of considering not just crash and site data but also human factors issues that are often the key contributing factors to crashes. It will also be useful to incorporate aberrant driver behaviors (such as impaired or distracted driving) into the analysis. In this regard, a key activity will be distinguishing driver behavior issues from human factors issues when considering countermeasures (see Chapter 4).

Finally, keep in mind that solutions (in the form of countermeasures or treatments) are not being sought at this stage. The focus here is on thinking like a virtual road user and identifying and understanding those roadway components that could contribute to confusion, poor visibility, misperceptions, high workload, distraction, or other potential road user errors at a particular site.

3.4.1 Collect Site Data

- Compile the data necessary to assess the traffic safety performance at the intended site quantitatively and qualitatively.
  - The three critical types of data needed for this process include crashes, traffic volumes, and recent projects that might impact crash potential (e.g., lane widening projects, horizontal curvature, or the installation of new sidewalks).

- Obtain crash data.
  - Crash data is commonly collected at three levels: crash, vehicle, and person. Crash-level data is the most summative and generally includes information describing the crash or facts that apply to all parties involved (i.e., time, location, and highest injury severity in a crash).
  - Each crash database has its intricacies and limitations—consider data quality.
- Compile volume data (including recent project site revisions).
  - Use volume data with enough information to distinguish important traffic patterns. For example, if an intersection with two-way stop control is being evaluated, it is important to know not just the total volume of the intersection but the major versus minor road traffic and any turning traffic.
  - The most recent volume data available should be used. If there was a major change in traffic during the crash analysis period, it might be prudent to use volume data reflecting this change for the appropriate years.
  - Any quality issues or known limitations of the crash/conflict data should be described.
- Account for roadway revision projects (e.g., lane widening, changes in horizontal curvature, installation of sidewalks, or new mailboxes and signs) that might have impacted safety performance. Projects occurring within the data analysis period need to be considered for their impact on traffic patterns and safety performance.
- Consider the role of deliberate, aberrant driver behaviors in the crash data, including speeding, distraction, and impaired driving. Chapter 4 may help practitioners distinguish between human factors issues and aberrant driver behaviors.
- The outcome of this activity should be a time-consistent collection of crash, traffic, and project data describing the safety, behavioral, and roadway data relevant to the site.

3.4.2 Review Site and Existing Conditions

- During peak and off-peak hours, visit the site during daytime and nighttime conditions. If a site visit is not possible, Google Maps Street View or Google Earth could be used. Conduct a qualitative analysis of existing roadway, behavioral, and human factors conditions at the site. Visiting the site at a variety of times will help facilitate an understanding of the conditions facing road users under a variety of circumstances. The purpose of these visits is to determine the conditions facing road users and potentially affecting traffic safety. Conditions may include infrastructure, human, behavioral, and operational factors.
  - Infrastructure–Focus on the built environment at the site. What is the state of the infrastructure road users are dealing with? Is the infrastructure operating/functioning as intended? Items to consider include pavement and sidewalk condition, sign and marking visibility, presence of dynamic roadway/roadside elements, drainage issues, shoulder condition, vegetation maintenance, properly functioning signals (including pedestrian signals), roadway/intersection lighting, differences, if any, in up-stream geometric or traffic control conditions that may impact user decisions, and so forth.
  - Behavioral and Human Factors–How are road users responding to the built environment and traffic within and upstream of the project? Items to consider include drivers' use of passing or turning lanes, line of sight issues (to both signal and other traffic control devices), bicyclists or pedestrians traveling along the shoulder, pedestrian mid-block crossings, and so forth.
  - Operational–How can drivers be better directed and informed to travel more efficiently and with less potential for a crash? Items to consider include large queues from turning traffic, traffic frequently blocking intersections, signal timing, non-conforming signing and marking, cues that might lead to road user indecision, and so forth. Where does the current design include TSM&O strategies as the countermeasures? Consider VRUs and factors

such as long pedestrian wait times at intersections, no pedestrian signals, limited cross-walks, permitted left turn signals, distances to cross the street, and so forth.

- These site visits are similar to Road Safety Audits (RSAs)—and may be conducted as informal RSAs.

3.4.3 Identify Crash Patterns and Contributing Factors

- Quantitatively describe the safety performance at the site by mode, year, crash type, and contributing factor through an analysis of crash patterns. Police reports are a key part of this, but may not be comprehensive enough for crash diagnostic purposes.
- Understanding crash patterns for the site is crucial for quantitatively assessing the site's potential for crash reduction. There are several ways to effectively summarize crash patterns, and there is no one correct set of tables or charts to develop. While the quantity, format, and style of the patterns are up to the designer or traffic engineer, it is important to describe the crash statistics clearly and completely by mode, year, and severity.
- Use the number of crashes and the count of injuries for the crash trend analysis.
- Develop a statement of significant patterns and findings based on the totality of the crash/conflict analysis. The state of significant patterns and key findings should focus on the more severe crashes and look for crash types and contributing factors where the severe crashes are over-represented.
- Some key questions to ask include the following:
  - What is the nature of the crashes/conflicts observed? Are there any discernible patterns between or among property damage only (PDO) crashes/conflicts and crashes/conflicts involving serious injuries or fatal crashes?
    - What do the most common crash types (e.g., rear-end collisions, run-off-road crashes, and vehicle-hit pedestrians) indicate about the relative contribution of road users, vehicles, and environmental issues to the crashes?
  - What are the most common contributing factors cited in the crash records?

3.4.4 Conduct Human Factors Evaluation

Chapters 5 to 8 present more detailed discussions of the role of perception-response time, expectancy, visibility, and workload/demand in crashes. The following is a summary of key points related to human factors evaluation.

- Review crash or conflict data summaries and the site visit results to identify possible human factors issues for consideration in developing robust, science-based safety countermeasures.
- A human factors evaluation of a specific roadway site should start with understanding the human factors approach to driving and road safety performance. Several data sources could aid this assessment, including PIARC (2012), Theeuwes and van der Horst (2012), and Campbell et al. (2012). At its core, this approach considers and accounts for road user needs, capabilities, and limitations in (1) the design and operation of roads, vehicles, and pedestrian/bicycle/transit facilities, and (2) the identification of causal factors underlying conflicts and crashes.
- The road-user factor most often includes capabilities and limitations related to expectations, visibility, workload/demand, and perception-response time. It may also include driver attributes that influence capabilities and limitations such as age, training, and road familiarity. The environment factor includes elements such as road geometry, traffic control devices, and the luminance levels of signs and markings. The vehicle factor includes automobile and truck components such as tires, brakes, or special safety systems.
- Safety performance reflects how well these components (i.e., road user, environment, and vehicle factors) interact and work together to support road users' full and accurate extraction

of information and understanding of environmental cues and emerging situations that lead to effective decision-making by those road users.
- Some key questions to ask include the following:
  - From the perspective of a road user (both the typical road user as well as a road user who may be older or impaired in some way), what might be some sources of confusion when trying to extract the most meaningful information (MMI) from the road geometry and traffic control information?
    - In general, is there consistency and meaning to the geometrics, signs, markings, and traffic control devices that road users rely on?
  - How might unique issues associated with vehicle type contribute to crashes or conflicts?
    - For example, does vehicle size play a role in how well the driver or road user can see signs, markings, and other road users, or how well the driver can navigate through a roadway with narrow lanes and no shoulders?
  - Are there any unique environmental and road conditions that substantially increase road user stress, comprehension time to roadway information, or response maneuvers to hazards at conflict points?
    - Examples may be short acceleration/deceleration lanes, unexpected roadside hardware placement, quickly narrowed lane widths, significant visibility restrictions, steep grades, and so forth.
  - Are there any unclear or misleading cues between the roadway and the user?
    - Such cues may be the lack of a timely presentation of geometric, signing, or pavement marking information, or a conflicting presentation of such information. Examples include using non-standard or non-maintained lanes or shoulders, less than standard sight distance for conditions, or less than standard distance for acceleration or deceleration of the vehicle or situations where the speed differential is more than 15 mph.
  - Consider not just the factors present at the exact time of a crash but also factors or events that could have occurred before the crash interactions.

At this early stage, it is best to generate a Modified Haddon Matrix (e.g., Table 5) that includes all possible factors impacting safety performance. Specifically, the matrix should include any factors and combinations of factors (interactions) that could reasonably contribute to the known or suspected opportunities for reducing crash potentials at the site under investigation. Broad considerations should include crash or conflict type, frequency, severity, and contributing factors, as well as on-the-scene observations of the facility and representative traffic movements (including pedestrians, bicyclists, and transit vehicles). In this regard, some interactions may be quantitative and very specific, while others may be qualitative and reflect possible impacts. As indicated in the matrix in Table 5, pre-, during-, and post-crash factors should be included in the analysis.

The diagnostic process should very much be considered to be an evaluative activity, as the fifth "E" (evaluation) should exist at every stage of the safety prevention process and not only toward the end of the process as part of countermeasure evaluation. Planners, designers, safety analysts, and so forth play different roles throughout the safety prevention process, and thereby the evaluative perspective of why the crash happened and how to select countermeasures is gathered and used as input at every stage.

3.4.5 Next Steps

The Modified Haddon Matrix generated during this process should yield several contributing factors that can serve as a starting point for design revisions or countermeasure selection.

Chapter 9 discusses how to link these contributing factors to countermeasures so that the countermeasures that are selected and implemented are more likely to address actual issues associated with a set of crashes; Chapter 10 provides a series of decision trees to aid the selection of specific countermeasures.

However, most users of this toolbox may benefit from additional information to aid and sharpen their crash diagnostic process. Chapters 4 to 8 provide more details on key human factors issues (i.e., mismatches between the capabilities and limitations of road users and the demands placed on them by a particular roadway) as well as focused diagnostic questions to assess these issues.

Key Concepts

1. Adopting a Safe System approach to diagnostic assessment will help the practitioner (i.e., designers, traffic engineers, and others) assess a broad range of driver/roadway interactions and incorporate a holistic approach to identifying the contributing factors to crashes.
2. This does not require a re-invention of crash diagnostics—a Modified Haddon Matrix provides a framework for diagnostic assessment that more directly considers all road users and the supporting social safety environment and is consistent with Safe System principles.
3. Looking at interactions as part of the diagnostic assessment process is crucial: most crashes (or conflicts and near-misses) will result from interactions among two or more of the individual factors. Therefore, identifying known or possible crash- or conflict-relevant interactions will be critical for identifying possible countermeasures.

CHAPTER 4

Distinguishing Between Human Factors Issues and Aberrant Driver Behaviors

4.1 Objectives

The objectives of this tool are to

- Describe the differences between human factors issues and aberrant driver behaviors as contributing factors to roadway crashes,
- Provide information that can help the practitioner distinguish between these two types of issues, and
- Improve the identification of applicable countermeasures to crashes caused by driver errors.

4.2 Background

Selecting countermeasures that improve road safety performance requires accurately diagnosing the factors that contribute to crashes. A review of crash data reveals that driver error is a contributing factor in approximately 93% of crashes (see also Singh, 2015; Treat et al., 1979). However, some of these errors primarily reflect disparities between inherent driver capabilities and features of the roadway's design (e.g., limited lighting), while others reflect illegal or unsafe driver behaviors (e.g., texting while driving, driving while intoxicated).

Roadway safety professionals and design practitioners may confuse the nature and mitigation of human factors issues versus aberrant driver behaviors. Such confusion can place more blame on deliberate violations and misbehavior than is supported by the crash data, rather than on interactions between (1) the demands imposed on the roadway's design and (2) road-user inherent capabilities. This approach can have the effect of leaving the real sources of driver errors on the roadways (e.g., limited visibility, high workload, limited time available to react) unidentified and unaddressed by improved roadway design and operations. For example, the Transportation Research Board executive committee described the components of an RSA and a Road Safety Audit Review (RSAR) that included a survey of state agencies that chose *not* to implement RSAs and RSARs, and one reason given for this decision is that officers from these agencies claimed that behavioral factors account for 85% of the crashes, so the tools would thus not provide a good return (Wilson and Lipinski, 2004).

Also, understanding the differences between human factors issues and aberrant driver behaviors is important, as the broader roadway safety community and individual practitioners apply the principles and practices of a Safe System approach to roadway design. A key principle of a Safe System approach is that humans make mistakes. Accordingly, the transportation system should be designed and operated to tolerate these mistakes (Able et al., 2021). Accommodating road users' mistakes requires having an accurate understanding of the underlying causes and true nature of those mistakes. In this regard, a holistic approach to countermeasures is to consider not just physical treatments that can be added to a facility to reduce crash frequency and severity; countermeasures can also take the form of exposure reduction (e.g., of traffic volumes, travel times, or travel distance). In addition, countermeasures can be defined in terms of both crash frequency and severity (e.g., rumble strips can reduce both total crash frequency and crash severity).

For example, consider a one-mile segment of a two-lane, two-way road in a rural area with the following design features and 5-year crash characteristics:

- No lighting
- Utility poles within clear zones left and right
- 55 mph posted speed limit
- No edge lines or centerline markings
- Head-on collisions or run-off-road crashes that result in either fatalities or serious injuries
- Key contributing factors that include nighttime driving, inattentive driving, and excessive speed

A diagnostic process for this site that is pre-disposed to focus on aberrant behaviors might conclude that driver speeding behavior was the primary cause of these crashes and would therefore identify countermeasures accordingly (e.g., to recommend increasing enforcement activities or increase the number of posted speed signs to reinforce the 55 mph posted speed limit). However, a diagnostic process that considers human factors issues informed by key driver capabilities and limitations might note that the relatively high speed limit and the number of "exceeding the speed limit" crashes, combined with the lack of lane-edge markings and lighting, create a strong likelihood of frequent lane departures. Such an analysis would likely recommend a very different set of countermeasures, such as adding edge lines, centerline markings, and/or lighting to improve delineation and visibility. Again, it is important to accurately diagnose the factors contributing to crashes before identifying and implementing countermeasures that will improve road safety performance.

4.3 Key Concepts: What Are the Differences Between Human Factors Issues and Aberrant Driver Behavior Issues?

Human factors issues and aberrant driver behaviors are both real and significant contributing factors to roadway crashes, but they can reflect different (1) driver motivations; (2) patterns of interactions between drivers, vehicles, and the roadway environment; and (3) approaches to countermeasure selection.

Human factors issues include contributing factors to crashes that reflect mismatches between the demands placed on the road user from roadway design and traffic engineering features and the inherent physical, perceptual, and cognitive capabilities and limitations of road users (see also Campbell et al., 2012). In a typical crash with human factors as the contributing cause(s), the driver is alert and attentive and follows relevant traffic laws and the typical requirements documented in state driver manuals. In the driving context, human factors issues reflect how road users interact with roadway elements, traffic control devices, vehicles, and other road users. Countermeasures that address human factors issues focus on shoring up drivers' limitations (e.g., an advance warning sign notifying a driver of an upcoming work zone reduces the information processing requirements on the driver by giving them an early notification of upcoming roadway conditions) or on improving the capabilities of a driver (e.g., rumble strips augment the driver's visual capabilities by adding a tactile and auditory cue that helps the driver perceive when a tire has exceeded the lane boundaries). In this example, a pattern of run-off-road crashes in which a lack of clear lane edges seems to be a contributing factor does not directly reflect bad choices or risky behaviors on the part of drivers; it reflects a road condition that may not adequately meet the driver's visual needs to maintain a safe lane position.

The World Road Association makes a similar distinction and refers to human factors issues as those "psychological and physiological threshold limit values which are verified as contributing to operational mistakes in machine and vehicle handling. It deals with general and stable subconscious reactions of road users and excludes temporary individual reactions and conditions" (PIARC, 2019a).

Aberrant driver behaviors include contributing factors to crashes that reflect deliberate violations of law or unsafe driving practices such as driving while impaired by alcohol, texting while driving, or driving unbelted. The World Road Association refers to issues such as personality traits like aggression and conscious violation of traffic rules; appropriate countermeasures include driver education, campaigns for influencing driving behavior, and enforcement (PIARC, 2019a). Several established sources describe and provide countermeasures for crash types resulting from such behaviors, including the NHTSA's *Countermeasures That Work: A Highway Safety Countermeasures Guide for State Highway Safety Offices* (Venkatraman et al., 2021) that focus on behavioral tools such as education, regulation/traffic laws, and legal enforcement. Table 6 provides some sample issues and behaviors associated with these two types of crashes and their associated countermeasures (see also Campbell et al., 2012; Venkatraman et al., 2021).

Following Reason et al. (1990), it should be emphasized that the distinctions between human factors and aberrant driver behavior issues are not always clear-cut and that these categories can sometimes overlap. For example, a crash involving an alcohol-impaired driver facing complex signage at a freeway interchange could reflect both aberrant driver behaviors (alcohol impairment) and human factors issues (increased workload and impacts on available perception-response time because of the signage). Also, speeding behaviors could be associated with roadway design elements (e.g., lane width; see Campbell et al., 2012) that may lead to higher speed

Table 6. Differences between human factors issues and aberrant driver behaviors.

Issue Type	Sample Issues/Behaviors	Sample Countermeasures
Human Factors Issues	Failure to meet road user expectations	Improve design consistency, add advance information signs
	Limited visibility	Improve lighting, add delineators, improve pavement delineation
	High workload	Reduce number or complexity of roadway signs
	Limited time for road users to react	Improve sight distance, provide longer yellow signal lights, add advance warning signs
Aberrant Driver Behaviors	Alcohol and drug-impaired driving	Communications: establish positive social norms that make driving while impaired unacceptable
	Speeding and speed management	Enforcement: publicized and highly visible enforcement of practical, sound, and broadly accepted laws
	Distracted driving	Outreach: inform the public of the consequences of using cell phones while driving
	Drowsy driving	Regulation: Graduated driver's licensing for beginning drivers that might include night driving restrictions, or hours of service for commercial drivers

selection by the driver, or they could reflect poor speed selection decisions/deliberate speeding by the driver. Finally, a single engineering countermeasure could apply to human factors issues and driver behavior issues; for example, rumble strips may support improved lane-keeping performance for drivers on roads with limited delineation and a history of run-off-road crashes, as well as improve lane-keeping performance for alcohol-impaired drivers.

Perhaps the earliest and clearest distinctions between human factors issues and driver behavior issues were made by Reason et al. (1990). They collected data from drivers that confirmed the distinction between what they termed errors (i.e., human factors issues) and violations (i.e., risky and unsafe behaviors). They found that while errors are generally unintentional and are accounted for by limits on the information processing capabilities of the drivers, violations are generally intentional and are accounted for by various social and motivational factors. Reason and his colleagues made clear that the boundaries between errors and violations are not always obvious and that both can be involved in the same crash sequence. Nonetheless, their work provides a framework for diagnosing crashes and selecting targeted countermeasures. Their work also highlights the central role that intentions and motivations play in assessing crashes and distinguishing between these contributing factors during the diagnostic process.

Several in-depth studies have examined the contributing factors to crashes and can serve to further explain the distinctions between crashes caused primarily by human factors issues versus those caused primarily by aberrant driver behaviors. In 1979, Treat et al. published a seminal report for the U.S. DOT and determined, from an analysis of over 2,000 motor vehicle crashes, that nearly 93% were caused in some part by human errors; more specifically, they identified improper lookout, excessive speed, and inattention as the top reasons for crashes because of driver factors issues (Treat et al., 1979).

Figure 5 from Chapter 2 above summarizes the results. As seen in the figure, while most crashes indeed reflect some form of driver error, a subset of these errors (approximately 57%) reflect primarily "driver-only" issues such as alcohol or impaired driving because of drugs or alcohol, road rage, fatigue, and distraction/inattention. Others (approximately 27%) reflect interactions, including roadway designs and traffic operation features that place demands on road users that may exceed their capabilities (i.e., human factors issues). Using more recent data from crashes documented through the NMVCCS, NHTSA investigated a sample of 5,470 crashes and analyzed the events and associated factors leading up to the crashes (Singh, 2015). The results related to the involvement of driver, roadway, and vehicle factors as contributors to these crashes are consistent with the results from Treat et al. (1979).

Wierwille et al. (2002) developed a unique taxonomy to describe driver errors, which included sub-categories such as limited knowledge, training, and skill; impairment; willful inappropriate behavior; and infrastructure or environment issues. These sub-categories highlight the need to consider not only human factors topics such as driver capabilities and limitations but also how drivers interact with the surrounding infrastructure features. For example, failure to yield at an intersection may be the general category that describes the crash type, but this type of driver error may be broken down into more specific components, like intersection features (e.g., unsignalized or skewed) and specific reasons for not yielding (e.g., visibility challenges, limited time to react) (Wierwille et al., 2002).

Using 2017–2020 data from the CISS (NHTSA, n.d.b) and 2010–2015 data from the National Automotive Sampling System (NASS) Crashworthiness Data System (NHTSA, n.d.d) and taxonomies that included those used by Treat et al. (1979) and Singh (2015; i.e., human factors, vehicle factors, and roadway and environmental factors), Dong and Wood (2023) assessed the contributing factors to crashes. Similarly to previously reported findings, their findings showed that more than 95% of the crashes investigated involved human factors or included a human error.

In over 50% of these human error-related crashes, aberrant driver behaviors such as speeding, alcohol-/drug-impaired driving, or distraction were contributing factors. Again, this suggests that a significant portion of crashes include a design or traffic control issue as a contributing factor.

Overall, these investigations into drivers' involvement in crashes demonstrate that crashes are a result of contributing causes from various environment, vehicle, and driver factors (such as driver inattention), as well as the interactions among these factors (such as roadway designs that place strong demands on the road user).

Key Concepts

1. Human factors issues and aberrant driver behaviors can reflect different: (1) driver motivations; (2) patterns of interactions between drivers, vehicles, and the roadway environment; and (3) approaches to countermeasure selection.
2. Identifying effective countermeasures to address road users' errors requires having an accurate understanding about the underlying causes and true nature of those errors.
3. Some errors reflect human factors issues—mismatches between the demands placed on the road user from roadway design and traffic engineering features and the inherent physical, perceptual, and cognitive capabilities and limitations of road users.
4. Other errors reflect aberrant driver behaviors—deliberate violations of laws or unsafe driving practices such as driving while impaired by alcohol, texting while driving, or driving unbelted.

4.4 A Diagnostic Process to Distinguish Crashes That Reflect Human Factors Issues versus Those That Reflect Aberrant Driver Behavior Issues

Figure 8 provides a general diagnostic process as well as individual diagnostic questions to help clarify whether a crash or group of crashes most likely reflect human factors issues as contributing factors or most likely reflect aberrant driver behavior issues as contributing factors.

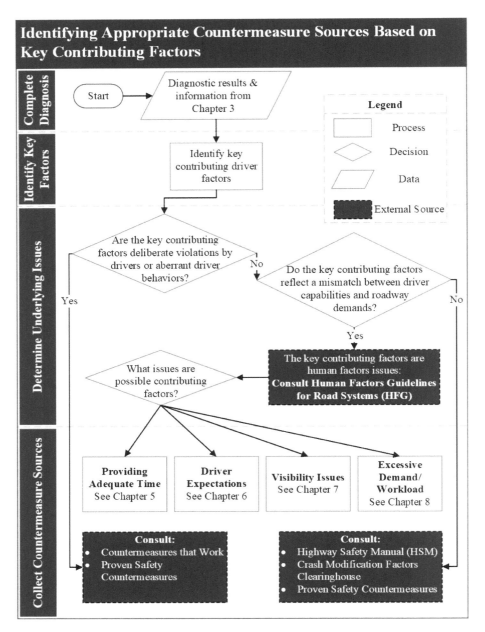

Figure 8. A general diagnostic process for identifying appropriate countermeasure sources based on key crash contributing factors.

CHAPTER 5

Perception-Response Time as a Contributing Factor to Crashes

5.1 Objectives

The objectives of this tool are to

- Describe the importance of time, and perception-response time (PRT) in particular, to road user performance and safety;
- Review the factors that affect driver PRT;
- Describe the relationship between driver PRT and driver expectations, visual conspicuity, and vehicle speed; and
- Provide diagnostic questions that can aid the practitioner in identifying factors that may reduce driver PRT in a given roadway area.

5.2 Background

A critical and common thread in circumstances that lead to roadway crashes is time—specifically, a lack of time for the driver to respond to an object in the roadway, a change in roadway characteristics, or a navigation demand. Time is not just a road user variable, it is also a design variable. Aiding the driver in ways that give them more time to perceive, decide, and respond to situations and conditions is perhaps one of the most direct ways that the roadway designer can improve safety performance. Probing both infrastructure and driver factors that relate to time and how they might impact safety supports improved diagnostic assessment of crashes and the selection of effective countermeasures to reduce crash potential. Time—and especially how drivers use the time they have—is crucial to assessing driver behavior in the context of crashes. The time drivers have to perceive and respond to an obstacle or object in the vehicle's path is called PRT, which is followed by the interval of time it takes for the vehicle to stop or change lanes (see Figure 9).

5.2.1 What Is Perception-Response Time?

PRT is comprised of four stages: detection, identification, decision, and response (Summala, 1981; Triggs and Harris, 1982; Olson and Sivak, 1986; Muttart, 2005). The PRT interval typically begins when an object of interest enters the driver's field of view and ends when the driver has just initiated the chosen response (e.g., begins turning the steering wheel or depressing the brake pedal) (Campbell et al., 2012). The four stages are as follows.

1. During the **detection** stage, the driver initially perceives an object of interest in the environment, which can involve seeing an object in their path of travel or hearing a noise somewhere in the distance.
2. Once the object is detected, the driver must **identify** it and determine whether it presents a hazard.

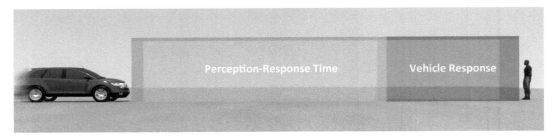

Figure 9.   General depiction of PRT and vehicle response intervals.

3. Next, the driver must **decide** what to do to avoid the hazard, if anything, such as braking, steering, or accelerating.
4. After the decision has been made to **respond**, the driver must initiate and carry out that action, such as moving the foot from the accelerator and depressing the brake pedal.

The four stages are not always present in every driving situation (e.g., there may not be a clearly defined moment during which the object is available to be seen by the driver, or the driver's initial identification may be erroneous) (Francis et al., 2020).

A large body of research involving laboratory and on-road studies has helped estimate approximate driver PRT values under a variety of situations. Although this range is wide (roughly 0.5 to 2.5 seconds), the data on PRTs can have significant utility in crash diagnostics and roadway design. AASHTO's *A Policy on Geometric Design of Highways and Streets* (commonly referred to as the "Green Book") recommends a design criterion of 2.5 seconds to include the capabilities of most drivers under most highway conditions, but actual PRTs will be situation-dependent (AASHTO, 2018).

For example,

- In a simple scenario where drivers respond to an expected situation during daytime (e.g., brake lights of another vehicle), PRT can be well under 1 second (Olson and Sivak, 1986; Fambro et al., 1998).
- When the situation is unexpected (e.g., a large plastic object hurled into one's path), PRT values can be as high as at least 1.5 seconds (Rice and Dell'Amico, 1974; Olson and Sivak, 1986; Fambro et al., 1998).
- During nighttime conditions, particularly in rural areas that are not well-lit, PRT values are closer to 2.5 seconds or higher (Summala, 1981; Triggs and Harris, 1982).

Therefore, driver PRT is determined by several factors that, under certain circumstances, affect one or more of the PRT components. Such factors include the driver's expectation of the situation or condition (e.g., an object in the roadway), its conspicuity within the larger visual field, the driver's visual capabilities, and the complexity of the required response. Although these (and other) factors can influence PRT, it is important to note that some are determined more by individual factors (e.g., age) or vehicle factors (e.g., handling), while others are more environmentally determined (e.g., lighting at nighttime). In practice, these factors act in concert, representing a complex relationship between drivers and their perception of the surrounding environment. PRT can also be affected by driver behavior issues such as impairment or distraction, but the discussion here is limited to human factors.

Various design resources conceptualize time differently and provide further guidance on the topic. The "Green Book" reviews some response time literature and provides formulas to calculate sight distance for stopping, passing, decision, and intersection visibility (AASHTO, 2018). The HFG (Campbell et al., 2012) has several guidelines related to response time and also summarizes much of the "Green Book" material on sight distance. According to the World Road Association's Human Factors in Road Design, drivers need 4 to 6 seconds to adapt to their normal driving program in case of unusual or complex information processing demands, apart from the standard response time for a sudden need to stop, which they call the "6 Seconds Rule" (PIARC, 2012). According to the authors, drivers would never expect a sudden change without an advance warning 6 seconds ahead. Given this, the authors recommend that when it is not practicable for critical points to be visible 6 seconds in advance, traffic signs or other advance warnings be provided to inform drivers of any critical point ahead (PIARC, 2012). Although this is a useful rule of thumb, it may not account for things like the speed of the vehicle or attention levels at a given moment.

5.2.2 What Factors Influence PRT?

Table 7 summarizes some of the driver and situational/environmental variables that can influence PRT (see also Campbell et al., 2012 and Muttart, 2005). Some of the more relevant factors identified in Table 7 are addressed in further detail in this section.

Expectancy, target conspicuity, and speed selection, which are three notable factors that affect PRT, are discussed in detail as follows.

Expectancy is a crucial component that can vastly impact PRT. In particular, if there is a sudden change in roadway characteristics potentially requiring a driver response (e.g., an upcoming sharp curve or grade, high-volume pedestrian crosswalk, change in posted speed limit, or freeway interchange), then it is reasonable to assume that a driver may not be prepared to quickly respond by braking or steering. Unusual roadway characteristics, such as left-hand freeway exits, may also contribute to increased PRT and crash rates. It is worthwhile to consider these variances in expectation in crash diagnostics and to implement advance warnings or signage in countermeasure selection.

The **conspicuity** of an object in the roadway will influence the driver's ability to detect it. Such failures in detection are associated with objects that are off-axis from the driver's line-of-sight, have diminished contrast relative to their background, and/or are small in size. Visual clutter is another roadway factor that can influence conspicuity and, therefore, PRT. Examples of visual

Table 7.   Examples of driver and situational/environmental variables that can influence PRT.

Driver or Situational Factor	Examples that May Increase PRT
Expectancy	Unexpected high-volume pedestrian crosswalk
Target conspicuity	Stopped vehicle without hazard lights on
Speed selection	Driving above the speed limit when cyclist darts out, even in well-lighted conditions
Target location	Pedestrian crossing mid-block
Driver fatigue	Overtired driver
Cognitive load	Talking on a cell phone
Age	Older driver
Contrast	Nighttime in a rural area
Visual glare	Increased glare from oncoming headlights
Familiarity	Novel or unfamiliar neighborhood
Visual complexity	Lots of signs, billboards, and lights (i.e., visual clutter) at a busy intersection

Table 8.   Distances (ft) traveled as a function of speed (mph) and time (sec.).

Time	15	25	35	45	55	65	75
1	22.0	36.7	51.3	66.0	80.7	95.3	110.0
2	44.0	73.3	102.7	132.0	161.3	190.7	220.0
3	66.0	110.0	154.0	198.0	242.0	286.0	330.0
4	88.0	146.7	205.3	264.0	322.7	381.3	440.0
5	110.0	183.3	256.7	330.0	403.3	476.7	550.0
6	132.0	220.0	308.0	396.0	484.0	572.0	660.0
7	154.0	256.7	359.3	462.0	564.7	667.3	770.0
8	176.0	293.3	410.7	528.0	645.3	762.7	880.0
9	198.0	330.0	462.0	594.0	726.0	858.0	990.0
10	220.0	366.7	513.3	660.0	806.7	953.3	1100.0

clutter include multiple, confusing, misleading signage, or a particularly complex intersection or section of roadway.

Speed is perhaps the most obvious influence on PRT; the faster an individual is driving, the quicker they will travel a given distance and the less time they will have to respond to a potential object in the roadway. Table 8 shows how far a vehicle travels as a function of speed and time. For example, a vehicle traveling at 55 mph will travel 80.7 feet in 1 second and 242 feet in 3 seconds. While speed limits influence driver speed choice, these are not the only or the most important influences. In addition to controlling speed by way of strictly enforcing appropriate speed limits (Richard et al., 2018), human factors research reveals that infrastructure elements (e.g., lane width, presence of shoulders, amount and location of vegetation on the roadside) can influence drivers' speeds, even subconsciously (Campbell et al., 2012). Even though direct speed information is available to drivers via their speedometers, drivers rely on sensory cues from the outside world (e.g., visual, auditory, tactile) to judge their speeds (Campbell et al., 2012). Although certain factors can lead to misperceptions of one's driving speed (e.g., rural roads without roadside trees can cause drivers to underestimate their travel speed; Campbell et al., 2012), research shows that certain countermeasures can have substantial impacts on actual driving speed. Specifically, drivers select speed using perceptual and "road message" cues. Understanding these cues and the messages they can communicate to drivers can help in establishing self-regulating speeds.

5.3 Key Concepts: How PRT Can Impact Safety Performance

Figures 10–12 provide an example of highway design cues that do not support timely and effective driver decisions and behaviors. In addition, the example highlights how time can interact with both expectations and workload as the driver approaches the decision point after passing complex and sometimes conflicting information from the highway design elements.

Figure 10 depicts the approach to an interchange that sets up some driver expectations for the upcoming interchange and depicts multiple destinations per sign/arrow. Note also that the "Exit Only" lane is indicated on the sign but not by the pavement markings, which can unnecessarily influence PRT.

Figure 11 shows that about 600 ft after the first set of signs, the next overhead sign content is inconsistent with the previous signs in both format and content. From the previous sign in Figure 10, it appeared that City Center would be in the same direction as Seattle (i.e., going North), but Figure 11 has no mention of City Center (or Beaverton). This inconsistency can cause additional workload as drivers attempt to reconcile the inconsistent information as the decision point approaches.

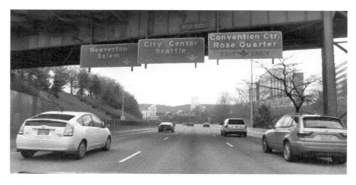

Figure 10.   Overhead signs set-up expectations for the upcoming interchange (photo by John Campbell, 2010; used with permission).

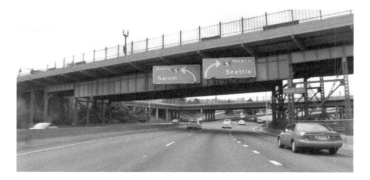

Figure 11.   The second set of overhead signs for the upcoming interchange that are inconsistent with the first set of signs (photo by John Campbell, 2010; used with permission).

Figure 12 depicts the signs at the interchange, about 500 ft beyond the second set of signs in Figure 11, which is the critical decision point for the driver. This decision point appears with limited warning because of the preceding overpass blocking the driver's view of the upcoming interchange (see Figure 11). The four signs at the interchange provide a great deal of information for the driver to perceive and comprehend (but which is once again inconsistent with previous signs) within a very short amount of time (approximately a second) before making a maneuver

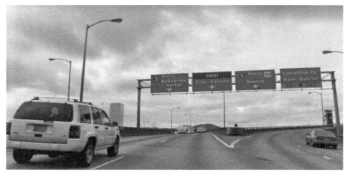

Figure 12.   The critical decision point for the driver where the interchange splits (photo by John Campbell, 2010; used with permission).

decision and then acting. If the driver is already in the lane that splits, this can likely be accommodated without any kind of abrupt maneuver, but if the driver needs to make a full lane change to go in the right direction (e.g., Seattle), sudden braking and steering maneuvers could impact safety performance.

Key Concepts

1. Aiding the driver in ways that give them more time to perceive, decide, and respond to situations and conditions is perhaps one of the most direct ways that the roadway designer can improve safety performance.
2. A large body of driver behavior research has helped estimate approximate driver PRT values under a variety of situations; most PRT values seen in the driver behavior research are between 0.5 and 2.5 seconds,
3. Driver PRT is determined by several factors that, under certain circumstances, affect one or more of the PRT components; these factors include driver expectations, conspicuity of detected roadway objects, and driver state (e.g., using a cell phone or not).

5.4 Diagnostic Questions Related to PRT

As summarized in this chapter, the amount of time available to respond to a changing driving demand or potential object in the roadway and how drivers use that time are critical components of roadway crashes. Having a better understanding of how concepts such as driver PRT and speed contribute to crashes is crucial to improving diagnostic assessments and ultimately preventing crashes with the implementation of effective countermeasures. When investigating a roadway crash (or crashes), the practitioner can consider different crash characteristics, keeping in mind how many seemingly subtle factors can have profound impacts on a driver's response time or speed. For example, it is crucial to consider the following:

- Can the driver see the upcoming object with sufficient time to react?
  - Specifically, is the encountered object in the roadway clearly visible (i.e., conspicuous) and in the driver's line of sight, or is it inconspicuous amid visual clutter and therefore detected later?
  - For nighttime, is the encountered object retroreflective and in the driver's line of sight, or is it inconspicuous because of factors such as limited lighting, low-beam headlights, headlamp glare, or physical obstructions such as trees?
- Has there been a change in the roadway, signs, or marking (such as a change in lane width, a new unlit pedestrian crosswalk, or a temporary sign) that may require the driver to make unexpected maneuver decisions?
- Does the signage that alerts drivers to upcoming situations and/or conditions appear in time for them to respond effectively?
- Is there advance signage to give drivers sufficient time to maneuver into appropriate lanes for upcoming highway exits, junctions, and transitions?
- Are the guidance messages on advance signage clear and consistent, such that drivers do not require more time to comprehend the messages?
- Can upcoming intersections be recognized by drivers in sufficient time from all approaches?

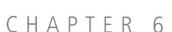

CHAPTER 6

The Role of Expectations in Road User Behavior

6.1 Objectives

The objectives of this tool are to

- Describe the importance of expectations to road user understanding of the roadway environment,
- Review the types of expectations that road users develop and where they come from, and
- Provide diagnostic questions that can help assess the extent to which expectations are being met on a roadway facility.

6.2 Background

Drivers use past experiences to anticipate the future and act in the present. Designing roadway environments in accordance with expectations is a crucial way to accommodate road users' capabilities and limitations, including their abilities to perceive and process information from the roadway in real time. When road users can rely on past experience to assist with interpreting communications from the roadway (e.g., signals, signs, and markings) and with the navigation and vehicle control tasks, they experience less demand because they only need to deeply process new or changed roadway information. Expectations are central to how a driver monitors, perceives, and interprets the roadway environment, makes decisions, and then acts or responds.

A driving environment that meets the expectations of drivers and other road users supports the accurate comprehension of roadway communications (e.g., signs, signals, markings), as well as effective and timely responses (Campbell et al., 2012). Mismatches between driver expectations and the roadway design can be a key source of misperceived and misinterpreted information and lead to "driving behaviors that are not appropriate for the traffic situation" (Martens et al., 1997, p.8). Such mismatches can be especially critical in situations involving time pressures and strong demands (i.e., a driver making a left turn at a signalized intersection with heavy oncoming traffic or a pedestrian or bicyclist deciding whether to cross at an intersection; see also Richard et al., 2006 for intersection examples). Roadways that are predictable and do not confuse or surprise drivers can allow them to plan for and anticipate decisions and required maneuvers efficiently, providing more time and mental resources to monitor dynamic elements that may be less predictable by nature, such as the real-time behaviors of other road users (e.g., vehicles, pedestrians, bicyclists).

Predictability is the key benefit to meeting users' expectations; predictability allows the road user to place a roadway into a predefined category that—in turn—dictates behavior. As Theeuwes (2021) puts it: "maximum information with least cognitive effort is achieved when categories map onto the perceived world structure as closely as possible" (p.5). In this regard, roadways that meet user expectations can function like a familiar "script" that directs and supports behaviors that are both effective and timely. Mental scripts are relied on to guide and support behaviors in many situations, such as eating at a restaurant, going to a theatre, or making a medical appointment. Navigating the roadways as a driver, bicyclist, or pedestrian similarly benefits from physical environments, sequences of required actions, and interactions with others that are predictable.

Expectations refer to a road user's readiness to respond to situations, events, and information in predictable and successful ways (Alexander and Lunenfeld, 1986). For the driver, expectations are closely related to the broader principle of design consistency. Design consistency is one of the most basic principles in human factors and system design. Consistency improves user performance because it facilitates the user's ability to predict what the system will do in any given situation; it provides rules that govern relationships between elements in the environment (e.g., signage and geometry) and driver responses (e.g., navigation and speed selection). The same underlying principle applies to other road users, such as bicyclists, pedestrians, and transit users.

Roadway designers and traffic engineers have long understood the benefits provided to road users through design consistency. Some examples of ways to provide consistency in roadway design include the following (Campbell et al., 2012):

- Recurring consistency in design elements such as lane width, curve radius, tangent lengths ahead of a curve, pavement surfaces, and roadside elements contributes to drivers' expectations about speed selection and lane position in curves.
- Route continuity, lane balance, sign placement, and sign content all impact driver expectations when navigating a complex interchange.
- Cross-section markings, guide signs, route markers, geometry, and sight distance are all key aspects of driver expectations on rural roads.

Martens et al. (1997) highlight the importance of design in supporting expectations as follows:

> The traffic environment should provoke the right expectations concerning the presence and behaviour of other road users as well as the demands with regard to their own behaviour. In order to reach this goal, clearly distinct road categories must be used, each requiring their own specific driving behaviour. (p. 8)

Expectations are also related to the positive guidance approach to roadway design; this approach reflects the road user's reliance on both long-term and short-term expectations to accurately predict, perceive, and respond to the immediate environment. Positive guidance is a critical heuristic that roadway designers and traffic engineers use to first identify site-specific issues and then to develop efficient improvements on their roadways (Lunenfeld and Alexander, 1990; Russell, 1998). A helpful principle provided by the positive guidance approach is for designers and engineers to consider the highway system as a holistic source of information—a real-time communications device—that is continuously sampled by road users for meaningful information.

Concerning traffic control devices, the positive guidance approach helps make roadways predictable and emphasizes assisting the road user with processing information accurately and quickly by considering the following design principles:

- **Principle of Primacy**–Determine the placement of signs according to the importance of information and present the information when and where the information is most essential.
- **Principle of Spreading**–Where all the information required by the road users cannot be placed on one sign or several signs at one location, spread the signage along the facility so that information is given in small portions to reduce information load.
- **Principle of Coding**–Where practicable, provide cues to the road user that help organize individual pieces of information according to more general rules. Examples of such cues include color and shape coding of traffic signs. These cues accomplish this organization by coding specific information about the message based on the color of the sign background and the shape of the sign panel (e.g., warning signs are yellow, regulatory signs are white).

- **Principle of Redundancy**–Communicate the same thing in more than one way. For example, the stop sign in North America has a unique shape and message, conveying the message to stop. A second example of redundancy is to communicate the same information by using more than one method (e.g., the no passing message can be presented redundantly using both signs and pavement markings).

The World Road Association (PIARC, 2012) describes the need to meet user expectations succinctly with the maxim "[n]ever surprise the driver" (p. 13) and defines the self-explaining road as "a roadway whose features 'tell' the driver what type of road it is and what design can be expected" (PIARC, 2012, p. 27). Such an approach to design helps guide the driver's response and provides visual cues that help the driver recognize and adapt to changes in speed, roadway function, or road user types (PIARC, 2012). Thus, designing the roadway with predictable features supports the development of expectations and a less-demanding task, which leads to driver responses (e.g., speed selection, the anticipation of transitions, glance behaviors that extract important information, and monitoring for hazards) that are matched to the nature of the roadway.

6.3 Key Concepts

Alexander and Lunenfeld (1986) noted that "expectancy is so basic to driving task performance and information handling, it should be considered in all driver-related aspects of highway design and traffic engineering" (p. 1). In general, drivers form expectations in several ways, including driver education and training activities, past and immediate experiences with the roadway facility that they are currently driving, and experience with different roadways that share design features with the current roadway. Two types of expectations can be supported by roadway design and traffic operations: long-term and short-term.

Long-term, *a priori* expectations reflect past experience with general types of roadway facilities (e.g., interstate highways), experience with a particular facility (e.g., the street a driver lives on), training, and even culture (Alexander and Lunenfeld, 1986). Drivers can use their *a priori* knowledge of a roadway section to focus their attention on aspects of the roadway most relevant to navigation and safety; this focus reduces the potential for overload and supports the development of learned patterns of behavior in response to specific roadway features or elements. For example, a driver approaching a stop sign at the end of a section of curved roadway may begin to prepare to stop even before the stop sign is visible based on prior knowledge of the sign and the roadway geometry. Pedestrians and bicyclists react similarly to familiar and predictable features along the roadway. Additional examples of long-term expectations include

- Using the color red to indicate high alert or *STOP* and green to indicate no threat or *GO*,
- Using the right-hand lane to make a right turn at an intersection, and
- Using, on freeway guide signs, destinations and arrows that match driving lanes.

Short-term, *ad hoc* expectations reflect in-transit, site-specific expectations corresponding to features such as road geometry, signage, presence of work zones, and land use (Alexander and Lunenfeld, 1986). Road users use *ad hoc* information to form new expectations about the facility to help guide the immediate task (e.g., driving, walking, bicycling). Some examples of short-term expectations include the following:

- When driving along high-speed sections of highways, drivers expect the same posted speed for the roadway ahead.
- A bus passenger or light rail user may benefit from an in-vehicle sign showing the next and upcoming stops.

- When curve warning signs are used ahead of several consecutive sharp curves on a rural road, drivers expect that future curves of a similar radius on the same road will be signed in the same manner.
- When a row of trees runs parallel to a stretch of roadway for a few miles at a set distance, drivers expect the same roadway/tree alignment on the roadway ahead.

Roadway designers and traffic engineers have long understood the benefits provided to road users through design consistency. Though tempered by design context and other local concerns such as land use, the importance of consistency is emphasized in design resources like the *Manual on Uniform Traffic Control Devices* (MUTCD) (FHWA, 2009) and the "Green Book" (AASHTO, 2018). For over 20 years, the FHWA has developed and maintained the Interactive Highway Safety Design Model (IHSDM) as a suite of software analysis tools for evaluating the safety and operational effects of geometric design in the highway project development process. The Design Consistency Module is one of five modules within the IHSDM and evaluates operating speed consistency through a speed-profile model that estimates expected 85th percentile, free-flow, passenger vehicle speeds along two-lane rural highways (FHWA, 2023b).

Seeing the roadway as a communications device is critical to producing roadways that are self-explaining, that is, roadways that produce safe driving simply through their design (Theeuwes, 2021). According to Theeuwes, this approach to design reflects the primacy of vision and visual selection in driving. It emphasizes how past driving experiences over a particular section of roadway bias visual search behavior when driving the same or similar roadway. Specifically, these past driving experiences help us learn and automate visual attention and responses to the environment through the selection of highly relevant information and the rejection of noise or distracting information. Road designs that are confusing and inconsistent violate expectancies and increase the likelihood of errors.

Charman et al. (2010) reviewed the literature on self-explaining roads and highlighted the importance of including physical features and cues in a roadway that help the road user identify the roadway as belonging to a particular category (i.e., functional class). Once road users understand the category of a particular roadway, they can identify the responses (e.g., required glance behaviors, speed selection) most appropriate for that roadway category. Charman et al. (2010) identified the following characteristics as supporting self-explaining roads and road user expectations by making categories of roadway types more easily distinguishable from one another:

- Unique roadway elements (i.e., homogeneous elements within a category and different from other categories)
- Unique responses for a specific category (i.e., homogeneous responses within a category and different from other categories)
- Avoidance of fast transitions going from one road category to the next; clearly marked transitions and changes
- Roadway elements (e.g., signs and markings) that define distinct categories, clearly visible under all driving conditions

This section concludes with an example that illustrates how upstream roadway elements can build expectations that can confuse and mislead drivers if the downstream portion of a facility is inconsistent with these expectations. The sequence of photographs (used with the kind permission of Samuel Tignor) in Figure 13 illustrates an example of design cues that can mislead drivers and contribute to unexpected situations. The photographs depict a two-lane arterial roadway crossing over a parkway that prohibits trucks. The first route marker (top photograph) shows the arterial roadway veering to the right. The first word sign (middle photograph), however, suggests that the arterial roadway is off to the left; the first line on this sign also suggests

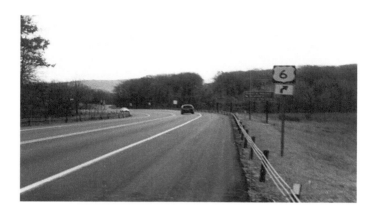

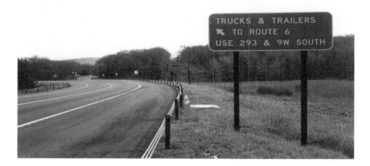

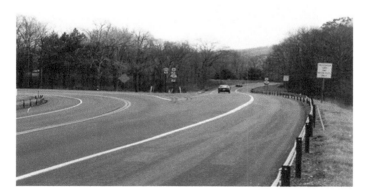

*Figure 13.   Example of roadway information
that could confuse drivers about vehicle guidance
requirements and lead to unpredictability and
unexpected demands (photos by Samuel Tignor,
2007; used with permission).*

that the sign is for trucks and trailers. From the skid marks near the gore (bottom photograph), road users are uncertain about whether to follow the road to the left or continue straight onto the ramp to the parkway. Especially for a driver unfamiliar with this section of roadway, the first two signs can create misleading expectations about the upcoming transition to the arterial roadway, leading to confusion and last-minute driver maneuvers.

Key Concepts

1. Mismatches between driver expectations and the roadway design can be especially critical in situations involving time pressures and strong task demands.
2. Roadways that meet user expectations and are predictable can function like a familiar "script" that directs and supports behaviors that are both timely and effective.
3. Design consistency improves user performance because it facilitates the user's ability to predict what the system will do in any given situation; it provides rules that govern relationships between elements in the environment (e.g., signage and geometry) and driver responses (e.g., navigation and speed selection).
4. Drivers form expectations in several ways, including driver education and training activities, past and immediate experiences with the roadway facility that they are currently driving, and experience with different roadways that share design features with the current roadway.

6.4 Diagnostic Questions Related to Expectations

Assessing violations of driver expectancies requires assessing potential surprises, changes, or clear violations of what a reasonable driver would expect at a particular site. This assessment serves as a first step toward determining if expectancy concerns exist within a facility. It may yield ideas for revisions that might address such violations and should include sections of the facility both upstream of the site under review and the site itself. The assessment should also reflect elements that could surprise drivers unfamiliar with the roadway and those that would surprise a driver familiar with the roadway. Some key questions include the following [adapted from Checklist E in Lunenfeld and Alexander (1990); and PIARC (2012)]:

- Are there any site-specific expectations that would have been formed upstream of a specific section of the facility (perhaps where there have been crashes) that (1) may have been violated and (2) contributed to the observed crashes? For example, consider the following:
  - Have there been any upstream changes to road type, lane/shoulder width, road surface, road lighting, shoulder drop-off, or cross-section?
  - Have there been any changes in traffic volume, traffic mix, or traffic operations?
  - Have there been any signing, marking, signalization, or other information display changes?
  - If the answer to any of these questions is "yes," consider if advance warning signs or other interventions may help to support driver responses. In many cases, such changes may simply require time for road users to adjust expectations.
- Are there any site-specific expectations that may have been violated? For example, consider the following:
  - At the site, are drivers surprised by key elements within the facility, i.e., roadway design and geometry, signs and markings, and visibility?

- Are changes in road characteristics, roadway alignment, or driving requirements communicated early and clearly by salient roadway elements (geometry, signs, markings)?
- As drivers enter built-up urban areas with more mixed road users (e.g., more pedestrians or bicyclists), does the roadway provide unambiguous cues to help the driver recognize needed changes in speed or a need to make changes in the driver's glance patterns to detect potential hazards?
- Are there any elements drivers might find unusual, perhaps some first-of-a-kind features?
- Are there any elements or maneuvers that might surprise drivers?
- Are there any changes in the site's operating practices; this could include new school zones or work zones?
- Are there any changes in the site's visibility characteristics (e.g., lighting, sight lines)?
- If any advance warning elements are present—are they inconspicuous or insufficiently descriptive?
- If the answer to any of these questions is "yes," consider if advance warning signs or other interventions may help to support driver understanding. As with the upstream changes, such changes may simply require time for road users to adjust expectations.

CHAPTER 7

The Role of Visibility
in Road User Behavior

7.1 Objectives

The objectives of this tool are to

- Define visibility and related characteristics as they relate to roadway safety,
- Describe the importance of visibility on driver performance,
- Describe how limited visibility in the driving environment can lead to errors and mistakes, and
- Provide diagnostic questions that can aid the practitioner in assessing the visibility concerns in a given roadway area.

7.2 Background

Visibility refers to the quality or state of being visible and relates to concepts such as conspicuity and sight distance. Vision is the primary source of information when operating a motor vehicle, with some researchers estimating that as much as 90% of information for the driving task is captured through the eyes (Hills, 1980). Studies of the visual behavior of drivers in real-world traffic conditions have found that drivers look at several important stimuli both inside and outside the vehicle to perform their tasks (Tijerina et al., 2004; Falkmer and Gregersen, 2005; Krauss, 2015). Whether or not these objects are visible to a driver at a particular point in time depends on features of the object (e.g., size, distance, and contrast with the background), features within the immediate environment that might block or obscure the object, and the attention directed by the driver toward the object.

The visual system uses a variety of cues to detect, identify, and localize objects in the environment. A primary cue that determines how quickly an object in the roadway is detected and acted on is that object's conspicuity. Conspicuity is defined by Krauss (2015) as "those characteristics of an object or condition that determine the likelihood that it will come to the attention of an observer" (p. 57). In other words, conspicuity refers to how noticeable or visible an object is. Some of the features that increase conspicuity include brightness and contrast (e.g., reflectorized traffic signs; Olson et al., 1992), color (e.g., the orange colors of traffic cones), location (e.g., objects in the center of view are more likely to be noticed than peripherally placed objects; Krauss, 2015) and size (Campbell et al., 2004). A driver's ability to select and act on even highly visible and conspicuous objects may be impacted by the amount and type of proximate visual information (e.g., pedestrians, other vehicles, signs, markings, buildings, planters, and so forth) in the immediate environment (Edquist and Johnson, 2008). Thus, the complexity and clutter associated with a visual scene impact visibility.

A driver's ability to respond quickly to an object in the roadway also depends on the distance available to visually perceive the object (i.e., sight distance; Campbell et al., 2012). Sight distance depends on scene illuminance and visibility, especially during nighttime conditions, as well as roadway design features such as vertical curvature. Pedestrian visibility is impacted by several factors, including lighting conditions, the size of the pedestrian, and the color/reflectivity of the clothing worn by the pedestrian (Campbell et al., 2012). Sight distance is directly related to the time drivers have to respond to an obstacle or situation ahead. The more visible the object or situation is ahead, the more time drivers have to perceive, decide, and respond. Conversely, the less visible the object or situation is ahead, the less time drivers have.

7.2.1 Why Is Visibility Important to Safety Performance?

As noted above, most of the information a driver uses is captured by their eyes. According to Tijerina et al. (1995a), a reduced visibility crash is defined as "interference, caused by low light or obscurance, with the capability of the road, other vehicles, or potential obstacles (including pedestrians) to stand out in relation to their backgrounds to be readily detected by the driver" (p. 1). Reduced visibility applies to both day and night conditions and conditions of fog, dust, rain, snow, or other atmospheric obscurants. Such hindrances to visibility may also be because of environmental objects restricting sight distances. Indeed, visibility is important to consider when developing diagnostic tools and countermeasures for roadway crashes, as low visibility increases the likelihood of crashes. According to Treat et al. (1979), one of the leading environmental factors related to traffic crashes is visibility.

A wide variety of categories influence visibility and how it relates to the likelihood of roadway crashes. These categories are not exhaustive but provide a glimpse into factors that play a role in rendering the roadway visible. The discussion focuses on topic areas that are important and relevant to roadway design and operations, especially those that contain features designers could modify to enhance visibility. For example, weather conditions and time of day are factors that cannot be controlled to mitigate crash potential. However, roadway signage and roadway design are determined by highway and traffic engineers and can be created to interact with uncontrolled factors to enhance visibility.

7.2.2 What Roadway Design Elements Affect Visibility?

In general, road signs, lane markings, and lighting are roadway-design elements that can significantly impact visibility, especially at night (FHWA, 2022a), and help address visibility limitations based on roadway geometry (e.g., sharp horizontal curves or vertical curves). For example, advance signage can inform the driver of upcoming limited visibility situations, and well-maintained retroreflective signs can improve nighttime visibility and reduce the risk of crashes by making signs appear brighter and easier to see and read from a distance. Similarly, well-maintained lane markings can make road curvatures more visible from a greater distance, thereby preparing the driver for unexpected curves. Finally, roadway lighting helps make roadways and surrounding areas and road users, such as pedestrians, more visible at night.

7.3 Key Concepts: What Are the Relationships Between Visibility, Vision, and Attention?

While visibility relates most directly to the quality of being visible, it is also closely related to drivers' visual abilities, as well as attention. Key aspects of drivers' visual abilities include the following:

- **Visual acuity**—The ability to see details at a distance
- **Contrast sensitivity**—The ability to detect slight differences in luminance (brightness of light) between an object and its background
- **Glare sensitivity**—The uncomfortable or disabling effects that light sources can have on nighttime vision
- **Peripheral vision**—The ability to detect objects outside the direct line of sight of the eye

- **Movement in depth**—The ability to estimate the speed of another vehicle by the rate of change of the visual angle of the vehicle created at the eye
- **Color vision**—The ability to see and distinguish colors in the visual field
- **Visual search**—The ability to search the rapidly changing road scene to collect road and traffic information

An alert and attentive driver will search for information to support trip navigation and second-by-second control activities, such as vehicle speed, level of braking, and steering. Campbell et al. (2012) describes this search for information as follows:

- Drivers scan the environment for the MMI about that particular road location and point in time.
- Drivers scanning patterns reflect the presence or absence of potentially challenging situations as they perceive them.
- Drivers are generally alert for both longitudinal and lateral challenges, such as other vehicles, pedestrians, animals, or objects near their planned path.
- Drivers develop an expectancy of the roadway based on what they previously experienced upstream.
- This searching and scanning process is continuous throughout the trip.

Figure 14 depicts this iterative visual sampling process.

7.4 Example of How Visibility Can Impact Driver Performance

The sequence of photographs in Figure 15 provides an example of roadway features that can reduce visibility and contribute to driver error. The photographs depict key parts of an 800-ft section of a two-lane rural roadway. The top photograph shows an upcoming horizontal curve, preceded by driveways on the right. Because of the close vegetation and sharp curves, there is limited visibility of vehicles entering the roadway from driveways, of pedestrians and bicyclists on the shoulder, and even of oncoming vehicles from beyond the curve. The middle photograph depicts a vehicle just entering the curve, with an additional driveway revealed on the left. This photograph also highlights the narrow shoulders on both sides of the road. Finally, the bottom photograph features a sag vertical curve, again with (mostly) hidden driveways to either side. Although visibility is the most obvious issue with this particular section of roadway, the presence of a relatively high driver workload (maintaining lane position plus watching for vehicles emerging from the driveways) and possible time constraints compound the demands placed on drivers, not taking into consideration additional visibility demands that would be associated with nighttime and/or inclement weather conditions.

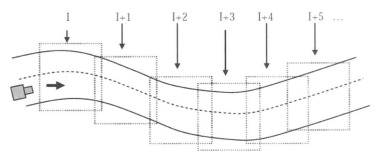

I = User scanning steps (vary in size)

Figure 14.   Drivers iteratively sample the environment to find the MMI (from Campbell et al., 2012).

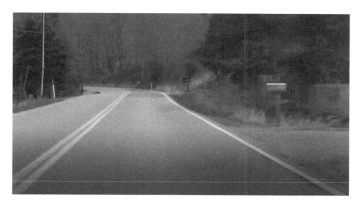

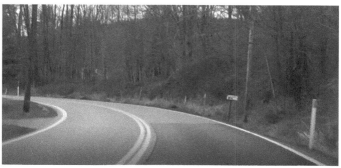

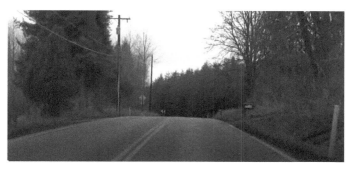

Figure 15.   Example of how reduced visibility can impact safety performance (photos by John Campbell, 2017; used with permission).

Key Concepts

1. Vision is the primary source of information when operating a motor vehicle; as much as 90% of the information for the driving task is captured through the eyes (Hills, 1980).

2. A primary cue that determines how quickly an object in the roadway is detected and acted on is that object's conspicuity, which refers to how noticeable or visible an object is.

3. A driver's ability to act on even highly conspicuous objects may reflect roadway lighting, sight distance, weather, time of day, and the amount and type of visual clutter (e.g., pedestrians, other vehicles, signs, markings, buildings, planters, and so forth) in the immediate environment.

7.5 Diagnostic Questions Related to Visibility

- Does the amount of sight distance available to drivers allow for safe driver responses?
- Are signs in place to aid road users in limited-sight distance situations?
- Are signs, markings, and traffic signals well-maintained, visible, and not obscured by fixed objects (e.g., vegetation), non-permanent objects (e.g., parked vehicles), or dynamic scene elements (e.g., moving cars, animals, pedestrians, bicyclists)?
- Are critical elements (i.e., intersections, driveways, curves, lane drops, and so forth) obvious and visible under both daytime and nighttime conditions?
- Does the geometry and surrounding environment support visibility around curves?
- Are there signs, markings, or lighting elements to support visibility where necessary?
- Will road users be able to see obstacles, guidance information, and information needed for traffic control and navigation?
- Are users seeing what designers think they should be seeing?
- Can users see what they need to see when they need to see it?
- Are there unnecessary traffic signs or other objects that may contribute to visual clutter?

CHAPTER 8

Task Demand as a Contributing Factor to Crashes

8.1 Objectives

The objectives of this tool are to

- Define workload and task demands as they relate to roadway safety,
- Describe the importance of demand (workload) on road user responses and performance,
- Describe how the demands of the driving task can lead to road user errors and mistakes, and
- Provide diagnostic questions that can aid the practitioner in assessing the demands that a facility places on road users.

8.2 Background and Key Concepts

Workload refers to the demands placed on an individual by a particular task, including effort, complexity, time requirements, and the nature of possible interference between concurrent tasks (Gartner and Murphy, 1979; Gawron, 2000; Angell et al., 2006). Consideration of the demands imposed on a user by a roadway facility is crucial to safety performance, as many crashes happen when the demands of the roadway environment exceed the capabilities of the roadway user. Table 9 provides some examples of situations that reflect this demands versus capabilities pattern and includes human factors issues and aberrant driver behaviors.

Although workload is a multidimensional construct, a useful shorthand for thinking about workload is to consider the time available to complete a task relative to the specific demands of the task; in other words, workload = time/task. While effort and time pressures are key aspects of workload, in the driving domain, workload is frequently described in terms of the following (Richard et al., 2006):

- Perceptual requirements (e.g., detecting and making sense of what is seen, heard, and felt)
- Decision-making/cognitive requirements (e.g., making decisions to go, stop, or turn; integrating what you perceive with things you know, such as rules of the road; or using your previous experience with a roadway facility to help decide what maneuver is appropriate)
- Psychomotor/response requirements (e.g., executing a decision, or taking action such as a driver changing their point of gaze to somewhere else within the visual scene, braking, or changing lanes)

These would include the demands placed on

- Drivers as they approach an intersection (e.g., seeking out the status of the traffic signal, maintaining lane position, and monitoring for pedestrians),
- Pedestrians crossing a roadway (e.g., planning a path and monitoring for vehicles), and
- Bicyclists riding within the lane or on the shoulder of a rural road (e.g., maintaining position, avoiding in-path objects).

Table 9. Examples of how the demands of the roadway environment can exceed the capabilities of the roadway user.

Situations that Create Strong Demands for Road Users	Ways that Road User Capabilities Can be Exceeded by These Strong Demands
Inconsistent signing regarding correct lane selection ahead of a complex interchange on a freeway	There may be a mismatch between formed expectations for lane position and actual required lane, under short time constraints—not enough time to change lanes safely.
Low levels of roadway lighting on a 45 mph arterial roadway with a pedestrian crossing mid-block at night wearing dark clothes	There may be insufficient luminance/contrast for many drivers to detect the pedestrian.
A vehicle making a left turn from a median lane into a strip mall driveway against heavy traffic from oncoming vehicles that includes bicycles in a bike lane	The driver of the left-turning vehicle is to perceive and track multiple hazards to find an acceptable gap, decide to turn, and then make the turn. This high workload can interfere with detecting other targets, like a pedestrian.
A speeding driver on the freeway (85 mph vehicle speed versus 65 mph posted speed) driving in the exit-only lane	The vehicle's speed may provide insufficient time to react to a suddenly appearing hazard, such as a vehicle attempting to reach the off-ramp through a series of sudden lane changes.
A driver looking down at their cell phone on a crowded freeway for extended periods of time	Reduced visual attention to the roadway can lead to a lane drift and a crash with another vehicle.
An alcohol-impaired driver approaching a line of slowing vehicles at a construction zone	Alcohol impairment can interfere with the driver's normal abilities to see, process, and react to slowing vehicles.

Driving even under the best of conditions is a demanding activity, as drivers are continuously performing several tasks at the same time while often moving at a high rate of speed. These tasks include visual scanning of the environment, perception and identification of task-relevant elements (e.g., other vehicles, pedestrians, traffic signs, and traffic signals), lane maintenance, and speed control. Critically, the driving environment is ever-changing, often requiring relatively high vigilance and attention to these tasks.

Driver demands associated with navigating a horizontal curve were included in the *Human Factors Guidelines for Road Systems* (Campbell et al., 2012) and can serve as an example of how consideration of demands can help understand how roadway design impacts performance. Figure 16 describes the activities drivers typically perform while navigating a single horizontal curve. This example shows that certain tasks—like maintaining speed and lane position while entering and following the curve—are more demanding and challenge the driver to pay closer attention to basic vehicle control and visual information acquisition. Also, since the analysis identifies the key information and vehicle control elements in different parts of the curve driving task, it can illustrate how and when driver demands are influenced by design aspects, such as placement of signs, nearby driveways, design consistency, degree of curvature, and lane width. In particular, identifying highly demanding (or high-workload) components of the curve driving task indicates where drivers might benefit from information regarding delineation or the elimination of potential visual distractions.

Assessing the impacts of task demands on workload and user performance has been an integral part of the system development process in other domains for decades. For example, the focus of the United States Army's Human Systems Integration program is to make sure that all fielded equipment and systems are designed to account for the capabilities and limitations

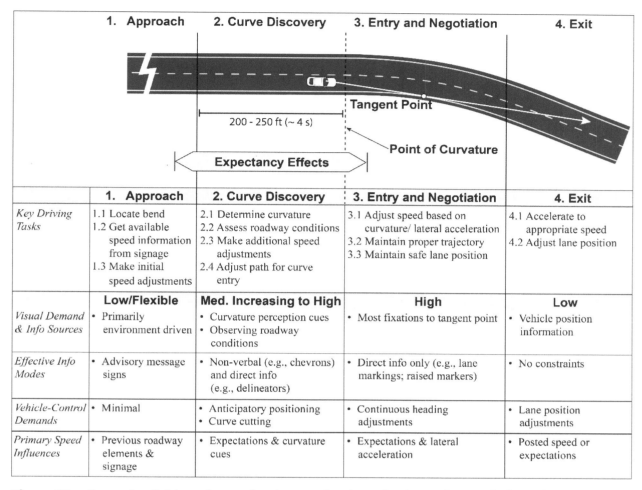

Figure 16.   Example of driver demands when navigating a horizontal curve (adapted from Campbell et al., 2012).

of users (United States Army, 2014). Rigorous assessment of users' tasks and their associated workload is a well-understood and routine activity conducted as part of the design and development of tanks, helicopters, military/commercial aircraft, and process control facilities such as power plants.

8.2.1 How Do Demand and Workload Contribute to Crashes?

As discussed above, when the demands of navigating the roadway exceed user capabilities, errors, mistakes, and crashes are more likely to occur. Designers and traffic engineers conducting diagnostic assessments can consider the ways that roadway design and operational decisions could impact driver workload and try to avoid demanding too much of roadway users. Research into the relationships between driver workload and the frequency and severity of crashes makes clear that high driver workload is a significant contributor to driver errors and subsequent safety performance. In a study that links such errors to workload, Wierwille et al. (2002) examined the specific types of errors that lead to crashes through a series of analyses and data collection activities. They cite numerous such errors linked directly to high workload—usually involving visual demand. For example, in the context of discussing driver errors made while turning left at signalized intersections, they note that higher approach traffic speeds, greater traffic densities, and large vehicles causing greater visual obstructions all make left turns more challenging to the driver. Specifically, there are more information-gathering points for left-turning drivers to sample, more vehicle-to-vehicle closing rates to estimate, and more chances of a missed detection. In the context of discussing errors made during merging maneuvers, Wierwille et al. (2002) note the following:

> A merging maneuver is considered to have a high level of driver workload associated with it; therefore, it requires a large amount of driver attention to complete safely. Drivers must be cognizant of traffic in the adjacent lane as they merge. In addition, drivers must judge the gaps between vehicles to be able to merge safely into the traffic flow, while monitoring any vehicle directly in front. A merging maneuver increases in difficulty when the speeds of the vehicles in the adjacent lanes are substantially different. Driver workload also increases when vehicles in adjacent lanes are weaving, that is, vehicles are switching positions between lanes. While a merging maneuver in and of itself has a high driver workload, decreasing the length of the merge lane greatly increases this workload, especially when traffic volume is high. (p. 172)

A concise summary of the problem associated with excess demand in the roadway was provided by Lerner et al. (2003):

> Drivers are frequently confronted with a multitude of information displays, which they must perceive, comprehend, and evaluate while they are simultaneously controlling their vehicles, monitoring other traffic, dealing with distractions, and navigating to a destination. In most metropolitan areas, one can readily find examples of freeway sites where within a few minutes of driving time there are dozens of elements of route guidance information, in addition to other information sources and distractions. The need for signing is frequently associated with complex traffic operations, geometrics, or potentially hazardous situations, so that the information load confronting the driver is often greatest when the demands of vehicle control, guidance, and crash avoidance also impose their greatest workload. When drivers are confronted with more information than they can process, they may decelerate severely or drive too slowly, make late or erratic maneuvers, take an improper route alternative, ignore critical information, fail to monitor other traffic, or have excessive episodes of eyes-off-the-road time. These behaviors have obvious safety and operational consequences. (p. 4)

In short, the workload imposed by infrastructure features on road users matters because mismatches between the demands imposed by the infrastructure and the capabilities of road users can lead to driver errors and crashes.

8.2.2 Identifying Task Demands and Workload Across Different Roadway Facilities

Workload is a challenge to measure, in part because it reflects characteristics inherent to the individual being measured—such as experience, ability, age, and so forth—but also because it depends on task- and environment-specific characteristics that influence demand and difficulty.

More detailed procedures are provided for measuring demands in Chapter 11, but—briefly—several researchers have developed workload assessment methodologies aimed at the safety practitioner. For example, Messer et al. (1979) emphasized the relationship between roadway features and driver workload, noting that workload increases

- With the increasing geometric complexity of highway features perceived to be potentially hazardous,
- With speed and reductions in sight distance for a given amount of work to be performed over a section of roadway, and
- For motorists who are surprised by the occurrence or complexity of geometric features.

Specifically, such situations will require more time and mental effort to decide on an appropriate speed and path. Using Messer's approach as a starting point, Krammes and Glascock

(1992) studied the statistical relationship between geometric inconsistencies and driver workload and found that driver workload measures could be good predictors of crash experience on two-lane rural highways (Messer et al., 1979). More recently, Tignor (2022, 2023) presented an approach to quantifying the frequency of infrastructure demands placed on road users by road designers. His focus is on elements of the infrastructure that users must interact with and respond to, including time between driveways, alternating curve and tangent renewal times, alternating horizontal and vertical curve renewal times, time spacing of warning and regulatory signs by direction, percent grades and grade travel time, and percent horizontal curve and travel time. Tignor's approach focuses on simple counts of these roadway elements—or workload "ticks"—to quantify workload as a function of roadway segments. Thus, he focuses on roadway elements beyond geometrics and simplifies the methodology for easier day-to-day use by the practitioner. Tignor's approach, in particular, focuses on assessing (1) static infrastructure elements within fixed roadway segments such as driveways, intersections, signs, changes in geometry, and transitions as well as (2) dynamic elements such as the number and movements of other road users, and typical vehicle speeds.

Access locations and associated access activities (e.g., entering and exiting vehicles, left turns and crossing traffic, freeway ramps, high-occupancy vehicle activities) are especially useful to account for as they are a chief source of dynamic conflicts and therefore increase task demands on the part of drivers who have to perceive and react to these access locations and related road user movements.

The nature and source of high task demands will vary considerably across different roadway types and driving conditions. Table 10 shows some typical roadway types and highlights features that could increase demands.

Related to time is the need to consider the effect of concurrent tasks on workload and the possibility of interference between competing demands on information processing resources. Road users have a finite amount of mental resources available to meet the demands of driving, walking, or cycling. These resources can be thought of as a "pool" of mental capability that is used to meet a variety of mental operations, from the visual processing required to comprehend a single road sign to the more complex processing required to extract meaning from a scene such as a crowded, multi-lane urban intersection.

This shared pool of resources is allocated across different tasks, modalities (e.g., visual and auditory), and processing requirements (Wickens, 2008). Interference between concurrent tasks reflects basic human limitations; for example, drivers cannot look at two separate locations in the visual field at once, and drivers have difficulties listening to navigation instructions while carrying on a conversation with a passenger. Concurrent tasks that "pull" from the same mental resources can interfere with operator performance on one or both tasks. This understanding of finite mental resources helps explain how very difficult individual tasks (e.g., making a left turn across traffic) can run into processing difficulties (e.g., high visual demand) and how multi-task performance is more likely to be hampered by performing similar tasks (e.g., looking at and manually tuning a radio while needing to monitor the forward roadway) than by performing dissimilar tasks (e.g., merely listening to the radio while driving).

In the driving environment, drivers often have concurrent and competing demands. For an example of competing for visual demands, consider a driver having to change lanes on a crowded freeway to reach an exit lane. The driver must balance the need to visually check traffic in adjacent lanes while visually tracking the location of the exit. From a response perspective, the driver may be making steering wheel inputs while adjusting speed. In general, higher demand is associated with multiple, concurrent demands that compete for the same mental resources.

Table 10.   Roadway elements that can increase demands on road users (photos by Samuel Tignor, 2021; used with permission).

Roadway Types	Elements That Can Increase Demands on Road Users
Interstate Highways	• High speeds can translate into reduced time to respond to conflicting vehicles. • High levels of visual demand—frequent glances to adjacent lanes are required to respond to multi-vehicle moving hazards (e.g., merge maneuvers, cut-ins, stopped vehicles ahead). • Conflicting moving vehicles could enter the road from the ramp. • Perceptual and decision-making demand is higher with smaller gaps (dense traffic) for merging and lane changing.
State Routes	• Curves and vegetation obstruct delineation cues and oncoming vehicles near a hill. • Potential for hidden driveways • Visibility/expectancy at intersections • Presence of bicyclists and pedestrians • Visibility/expectancy is questionable at unexpected intersections. • Possible conflicts at the crest of a hill and turning road • Guardrail close to roadway restricts possible escape path
Rural Roads	• Potential vehicles, pedestrians, or bikes at or beyond the crest • Narrow lane widths on each side of the road • Potential for hidden driveways • Narrow roadway with no centerline plus narrow shoulders • An unexpected vehicle can enter the road from a driveway.
Urban	• Highly dynamic traffic elements—stopping and turning vehicles, many bicycles, scooters, and pedestrians are cramped into the intersection. • Challenging road user guidance and navigation in a dense-visual environment • Visibility of other road users (e.g., the two bike lanes in the center of the street are hard to perceive, and pedestrians may be blocked by other vehicles) • Two-way traffic on a cross street • Traffic signals and signs must be perceived and comprehended.
City Center	• A mix of road users—pedestrians, bicyclists, scooters—often in unexpected locations • Many traffic control devices—traffic signals, signs • Dynamic traffic elements—stopping and turning vehicles • Challenging road user guidance and navigation in a dense-visual environment • Extremely limited visibility/expectancy throughout the street • Large trucks and buses block users' visibility and mobility. • Traffic signals, signs, and pavement markings are blocked by queued vehicles. • User workload is extremely high for all modal users.

Individual characteristics play a role in workload considerations as well. Consider an older driver with reduced perceptual capabilities (e.g., difficulties seeing at night) or reduced physical capabilities (e.g., slower braking response). Certain situations might place higher demands on that older driver, leading to a higher workload relative to a younger driver. However, differences in skills and abilities across drivers play a role as well. A highly-skilled driver may experience less workload than a lower-skilled driver when navigating a particular section of roadway for the first time.

Overall, whether because of task difficulty, time demands, interference between competing mental resources, or individual differences (or some combination of these factors), consideration of the demands a facility places on road users is key to evaluating safety performance. Road-user errors are more likely to occur when the demands of the roadway environment exceed the capabilities of the roadway user. While overload is the most common problem faced by road users (as seen in the examples in Table 10), this mismatch between demands versus capabilities can occur when the demands are too high or too low. Figure 17 shows the general relationship between task performance and task demands. As seen, performance can be impacted when the workload is high (e.g., having to read many critical guidance signs in a short period) but also when it is too low (e.g., driving along a straight highway with little traffic for long periods) if road users become bored, unengaged, or complacent.

8.2.3 Example of How High Workload Can Impact Safety Performance

The sequence of photographs in Figure 18 provides an example of roadway features at a freeway offramp that can lead to high levels of driver workload and impact safety performance. The signs depicted in the top photograph indicate that either of the two right-most lanes may be used for both Blue Oaks Boulevard and Washington Boulevard. The middle photograph, however, shows that, of these two lanes, Washington Boulevard can only be accessed by the lane on the left. The third photograph depicts some additional signage to the right and a final set of overhead signs to be comprehended if the driver needs to decide about going westbound or eastbound on Blue Oaks Boulevard. Overall, this offramp presents a driver with a great deal of information to perceive, comprehend, and react to, which may be challenging for a driver unfamiliar with this location to process. This example combines issues with setting up incorrect expectations (the message on the first sign) with strong demand in the form of information overload through many signs presented in a short period.

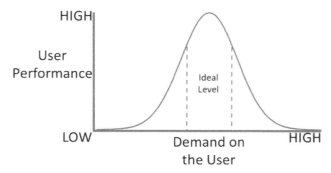

Figure 17. General relationships between performance and task demands.

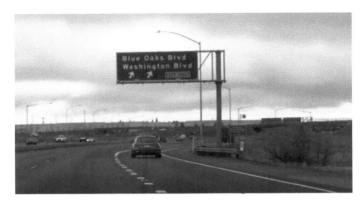

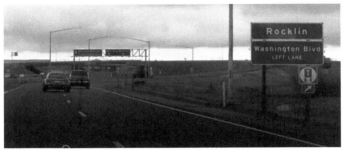

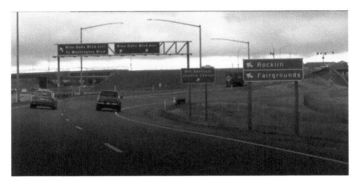

Figure 18.   Example of potentially high workload (or high demand) driving resulting from complex and conflicting signage (photos by Keith Harrison, 2014; used with permission).

Key Concepts

1. Many crashes happen when the demands of the roadway environment exceed the capabilities of the roadway user.
2. A useful shorthand for thinking about workload (or demand) is to consider the time available to complete a task relative to the specific demands of the task; in other words, workload = time/task.
3. Practitioners conducting diagnostic assessments can consider the ways that roadway design and operational decisions could impact driver workload and try to avoid demanding too much of roadway users.

8.3 Diagnostic Questions Regarding Demand and Workload

- Consider all demands within the context of available time and speed—do posted speeds allow for enough time to meet individual demands?
- From the crashes/conflicts observed, are there any patterns that would indicate that workload was a contributing factor? Are there any discernible patterns between or among crashes/conflicts and crashes/conflicts involving serious injuries or fatal crashes that could relate to demand?
- Within the facility, are there any possible sources of confusion for a road user trying to extract information from the road geometry and traffic control information? Specifically, is there consistency and meaning to the collective use of geometrics, signs, markings, and traffic control devices that road users rely on?
- Taking into consideration user tasks and subsequent workload demands, are there any activities that suggest the presence of competing roadway demands that might unduly increase perceptual, cognitive, or psychomotor requirements for the road user?
- Are there any unique environmental or road conditions that substantially increase road user stress, time to perceive and extract roadway information, or time to respond to hazards at conflict points (e.g., short acceleration/deceleration lanes, unexpected roadside hardware placement, quickly narrowed lane widths, significant visibility restrictions, steep grades, and so forth)?
- Are crashes occurring at or near access points (e.g., consider locations of driveways in relation to the intersections, turning traffic, and sight obstructions at driveways)? [Harwood et al. (2010)]
- Are dilemma-zone crashes occurring at intersections because drivers might be having difficulty making stop/go decisions? [Harwood et al. (2010)]
- Are crashes occurring because of turning drivers failing to detect pedestrians, bicyclists, or scooters? Are there environmental elements at these locations that could be causing distractions? Do pedestrians walk onto the road while waiting to cross moving transit or seeking to catch buses? [PIARC (2019b)]
- Are signs and markings collectively clear, unambiguous, and consistent? [PIARC (2019b)]
- Have unnecessary signs been avoided or eliminated? [PIARC (2019b)]
- Are signs clearly visible when other roadway noise is present (community banners, advertisements, vegetation)?
- Are the movements for all road users, including VRUs, guided clearly and easy to understand? [PIARC (2019b)]

CHAPTER 9

Linking Contributing Factors to Countermeasures

9.1 Objectives

The objectives of this tool are to

- Describe the importance of linking countermeasures to the underlying contributing factors of relevant crashes,
- Provide a process for identifying, prioritizing, and evaluating countermeasures that are linked to contributing factors, and
- Provide examples of key crash types, representative countermeasures for these crash types, and descriptions of how these countermeasures aid road users.

9.2 Background

Roadways are communication devices, and they are at all times communicating a host of messages to the road user. Sometimes these messages are helpful and intended by the roadway designer, and sometimes not. Countermeasures can improve how the roadway designer communicates with the road user and can decrease the crash frequency or severity at a particular site. As noted in previous chapters of this report, many crashes happen when the demands of the roadway environment exceed the capabilities of the roadway user. In this regard, it is important to recognize that roadway countermeasures operate within this demand versus capabilities framework. Specifically, effective countermeasures decrease the demands placed on the road user and/or augment the road user's capabilities in some fashion. Accordingly, countermeasures are selected in a manner that links their features and benefits to the underlying contributing factors and human factors issues observed within the crash data or the facility itself. Chapter 4 distinguishes between human factors issues and aberrant driver behavior issues. Many countermeasures with proven effectiveness can be useful for both kinds of issues. For example, countermeasures that reduce vehicle speeds can address both deliberate speeding as well as giving non-speeding drivers more time to respond to unexpected situations and/or conditions. Similarly, countermeasures that generally improve the visibility of pedestrians may offer particular benefits to distracted drivers by increasing pedestrian conspicuity.

9.3 Key Concepts

The purpose of this discussion is not to recommend specific countermeasures, but to briefly present a process for identifying and selecting countermeasures and to show how frequently recommended countermeasures impact road users' perception and performance. Chapter 8: Countermeasure Selection of the HSM (AASHTO, 2010), discusses countermeasure identification and selection in the context of the larger roadway safety management process and—combined with the HSM/HFG Primer (Campbell et al., 2018)—should be considered a key source for this process.

Countermeasure identification, prioritization, and selection can consider user behaviors or information needs that reflect functional considerations (i.e., position and type of service being provided by roadways) as well as context considerations (i.e., how the roadway fits into and serves the community and multimodal needs and issues).

9.3.1 Overview and General Process

Discussion regarding the countermeasure identification and selection process picks up where Chapter 3 left off, with a partially completed Modified Haddon Matrix, developed by John Milton and Ida van Schalkwyk of the Washington State Department of Transportation and used with their kind permission. As with Chapter 3, the discussion is adapted from the HSM/HFG Primer (Campbell et al., 2018) that was developed to provide the practitioner with information from both the HSM and the HFG to aid in assessing the contributing factors to crashes and in selecting countermeasures.

Figure 19 illustrates this part of the process and is primarily intended to emphasize the importance of linking countermeasure identification and selection to specific human factors issues (as well as driver behavior issues) identified during the diagnostics process.

With a populated Modified Haddon Matrix, there is a process that could be used to identify and select appropriate countermeasures. While this process focuses on the decision trees in Chapter 10 of this toolbox and the HSM and the HFG as key sources for safety countermeasures, there are many additional sources that can and should be consulted when looking for countermeasures. These include sources published by the U.S. DOT, such as behavioral countermeasures found in NHTSA's Countermeasures that Work publications (Venkatraman et al., 2021):

- **Consult Chapter 10**
  - Chapter 10 provides a series of decision trees to help designers and traffic engineers select countermeasures that address target crash and facility types. Practitioners can select from a series of decision trees that lead the analyst through diagnostic questions to help identify countermeasures that could potentially address crash-contributing factors associated with the crash pattern of interest.

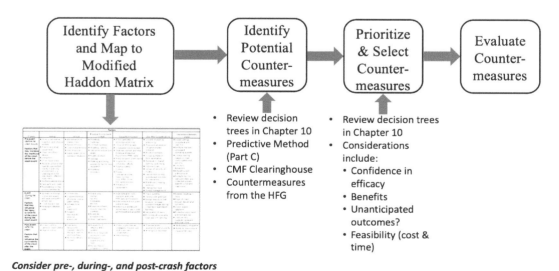

Consider pre-, during-, and post-crash factors

Figure 19.   Incorporating the Safe System approach into the countermeasure identification and selection process.

- **Identify Potential Countermeasures from the Highway Safety Manual**
  - Using the Predictive Method (Part C of HSM; AASHTO, 2010)
    - The predictive method employs safety performance functions (SPFs) to estimate the predicted crash frequencies for a network, segment, or particular site for specific base conditions. The HSM breaks the predictive method into an 18-step process, as summarized in a flowchart in HSM Figure C-2.
    - The following steps highlight the key methods in comparing treatments through the predictive method:
      - Predictive method Step 9–For the selected site, determine and apply the appropriate SPF for the site's facility type and traffic control features.
      - Predictive method Step 10–Apply appropriate Part C Crash Modification Factors (CMFs) to the results of the SPF to adjust the predicted average crash frequency to site-specific geometric design and traffic control features.
      - Predictive method Step 11–Apply calibration factors to the results of Step 10 as appropriate for the jurisdiction and time period of the analysis.
      - Predictive method Step 17–Determine if there is an alternative design, treatment, or forecast annual average daily traffic to be evaluated, and conduct alternative analysis as needed.
      - Predictive method Step 18–Evaluate and compare results.
    - To aid in the predictive method process, spreadsheet-based tools and additional guidance for the HSM are available for use with rural two-lane, two-way roads, rural multilane highways, suburban arterials, and urban arterials (AASHTO, 2010). These tools guide users through the application of SPFs, CMFs, and calibration factors for individual sites.
- **Identify Potential Countermeasures from the HFG**
  - Create a list of HFG contents (i.e., solutions, countermeasures, and design options; Campbell et al., 2012) corresponding to design characteristics or crash reduction opportunities within the road system. From the results of the Modified Haddon Matrix, consider especially pre-crash factors that reflect interactions between the road user and the infrastructure, and identify
    - Relevant road user needs, capabilities, or limitations;
    - Relevant road user perception or performance issues;
    - Specific HFG recommendations, countermeasures, or design options; and
    - Relevant data sources or research studies that could support specific design changes or enhancements.
  - This review of the HFG should yield a succinct summary of key road user issues, specific recommendations, countermeasures, or design options from the HFG, and any related information that will support a robust safety solution.
- **Prioritize and Select Countermeasures**
  - Develop a prioritized list of potential countermeasures to address the contributing factors identified through the diagnostic process. As noted throughout this toolbox, key resources could include Proven Safety Countermeasures (FHWA, n.d.d), the CMF Clearinghouse (FHWA, n.d.b), the HSM (AASHTO, 2010) and the HFG (Campbell et al., 2012). However, to get the most value out of these resources, the options and countermeasures provided by each document must be collated, compared, and considered as part of the prioritization process. See Chapter 10 for countermeasure options and trade-offs for a range of facilities and crash types.
  - The reviews will likely yield several countermeasure options and several general issues to consider. When selecting countermeasures, it is important to understand the road, crash types, volume restraints, and other factors under which the CMF was developed. In some cases, looking through such factors alone may eliminate CMFs from the selection. In most cases, there will still be multiple CMFs that appear to satisfy the site conditions and project requirements.

– To achieve a vetted and reliable project priority list, the following characteristics are considered for each of the previously identified potential countermeasures.

  ▪ **Degree of confidence**—Many potential countermeasures have multiple associated crash reductions. The selection of a particular CMF or calibration factor may play an important part in determining the overall crash reduction potential of the treatment. In particular, it is important to consider the quality and applicability of individual research studies supporting CMFs. It is strongly recommended that each treatment be evaluated for a degree of confidence based on the assumptions and engineering judgment used in the analysis.

  ▪ **Benefits**—What are the benefits of the solution? Is the potential crash reduction ample enough to justify the project or project changes?

  ▪ **Change**—Will there be a change in traffic, pedestrian, or bicycle volume at the site, which could lead to additional crashes in that mode because of increased exposure (e.g., will pedestrian traffic increase because of more reliable crossing signals, or are there no expected changes at all).

  ▪ **Conflicts**—Does the project create any built, operational, or road user problems with the existing area (e.g., will driveways' entries/exits become additional elements that could conflict with residents/businesses/bikes/pedestrians/less-mobile individuals using the road)?

  ▪ **Feasibility**—Is the potential solution cost and time appropriate and does it provide benefits for the expenditure? This does not necessarily include a full cost-benefit analysis of each potential solution.

– There is no defined process for synthesizing the results from both the HSM, the HFG, and other sources of countermeasures into a set of perfect countermeasures. Prioritizing the identified countermeasures requires comparing the potential countermeasures offered by each source to the details of the crash sites/situation at hand. Specific questions might include the following:

  ▪ What is the alignment between the engineering countermeasures(s), the crash patterns, contributing factors identified in the diagnosis, and the human factors assessment?

    ♦ Do the identified countermeasures/solutions seem reasonable given the crash data?

    ♦ Do they seem appropriate for the site and the general driving conditions?

    ♦ Will the countermeasures affect other modes of transportation negatively (transit, bicyclists, pedestrians, motorcyclists, and so forth); specifically, what are the trade-offs for these user groups?

  ▪ How do the tools and guidance from each source (the HSM and the HFG) relate to or complement one another?

    ♦ Is there consistency across the information provided by the HSM and the HFG? Well-supported guidance from both sources can provide a strong argument for solutions.

    ♦ Is more than a single countermeasure appropriate for the situation?

    ♦ How well would multiple countermeasures address the identified factors that seem to be contributing to crashes?

  ▪ Given the overall situation, what guidance from all sources seems the most feasible from a safety, implementation, and cost perspective?

• **Evaluate Countermeasures**

  – The purpose of a safety effectiveness evaluation is to determine the actual impacts of a project after it has been completed at a site. It might also be useful to evaluate a counter-measure at a single site before multi-site implementation and to help provide data for future decisions. Countermeasure evaluation typically includes a statistical comparison of crashes for a period before and after the project is completed. Often, the effectiveness evaluation must be conducted several years after the project is completed to allow for possible impacts to occur and for sufficient data to be obtained. Conducting an effectiveness evaluation will help guide future projects and improve project prioritization. Conducting evaluations (the fifth "E" of safety) to aid the selection and design of countermeasures is critical to improving safety performance.

- While an evaluation of effectiveness is strongly recommended, the process to do so is a field of its own, and practitioners should consult additional research for guidance; potential resources include the following:
  - The Crash Modification Factor Clearinghouse recommendations for developing CMFs (FHWA, n.d.b)
  - *Observational Before-After Studies in Road Safety* (Hauer, 1997)
  - The *FHWA Highway Safety Improvement Program Manual,* which has an entire section on how to go about such studies (FHWA, 2010)
  - The FHWA's evaluation guide, Highway Safety Improvement Program (HSIP) Evaluation Guide (Gross, 2017), which includes methods, data requirements and other aids associated with different types of evaluations

Also, Pullen-Seufert and Hall (2008) provide a seven-step process for evaluating highway safety programs and countermeasures, as follows (additional discussion for each of these steps is provided in Chapter 1):

1. Identify the problem.
2. Develop reasonable objectives.
3. Develop a plan for measuring results.
4. Gather baseline data.
5. Implement your program.
6. Gather data and analyze results.
7. Report results.

The following subsections provide countermeasure information for four types of crashes that account for a significant number of overall crashes in the United States: road departure, pedestrian, work zone, and intersection crashes. Roadway departure, intersection, and pedestrian crashes in particular are a consistent focus of the FHWA's HSIP. For each of the crash types, the following subsections include a brief review of the crash data, a summary of known contributory factors to crashes, and a list of typical countermeasures and how these countermeasures help road users, that is, how they decrease the demands placed on the road user and/or augment the road user's capabilities.

9.3.2 Road Departure Crashes

Motor vehicle crashes in which a vehicle departs its lane of travel, leaves the roadway, and strikes other objects or overturns account for approximately 64% of all single-vehicle crashes (Liu and Ye, 2011) and around 70% of all fatal single-vehicle crashes (Liu and Subramanian, 2009) in the United States. In-depth analyses of real-world crash and near-crash data have identified critical reasons—which describe the immediate reason for the vehicle running off the road but do not necessarily convey the cause or assignment of fault—and contributing factors to such crashes. The crashes can occur on straight, rural roads and can be influenced by a variety of driver-related factors, including overcompensation and imprecise directional control of the vehicle, falling asleep, inattention, and distraction (Pomerleau et al., 1999; McLaughlin et al., 2009).

9.3.2.1 Contributing Factors to Road Departure Crashes

Despite the range of possible contributing factors to run-off-road crashes, existing research has consistently identified inattention and/or fatigue/drowsiness as primary contributory factors for these events. For example, analysis of NHTSA's Fatality Analysis Reporting System (FARS) data from the 1990s and early 2000s identified several vehicle, environmental, and driver-related contributors, but driver fatigue was prominent as the most frequently involved factor (NHTSA, n.d.c). A sleepy driver was found to be more likely (more than three times the odds) to be involved in a road departure crash than an alert driver (Liu and Subramanian, 2009). More in-depth examination of run-off-road crashes has reported similar findings. In an analysis of run-off-road crashes from the NMVCCS database, Liu and Ye (2011) reported that, of all the contributing factors identified, inattention and fatigue were the most influential, increasing crash potential by odds of 3.7 and 3.5, respectively. However, these driver responses were not the only contributing factors identified; others included overcompensation (13.6% of run-off-road crashes), imprecise directional control (12%), and driving too fast for a curve (10.5%).

9.3.2.2 Typical Countermeasures and How They Aid Road Users

A variety of countermeasures have been developed to help drivers maintain their lane positions and avoid and/or mitigate exceeding the lane boundaries. Table 11 highlights some of these countermeasures and explains how they help road users by reducing the demands of the lane maintenance task and/or augmenting drivers' capabilities.

9.3.3 Pedestrian Crashes

In 2021, there were 7,388 pedestrians killed in traffic crashes; this reflects a 12.5% increase from 6,565 pedestrian fatalities in 2020 (NCSA, 2023a). In 2021, pedestrians accounted for

Table 11. Example countermeasures for road departure crashes and how they aid road users (adapted from Campbell et al., 2012).

Countermeasure	How the Countermeasure Helps Road Users
Rumble strips (e.g., shoulder, edge-line, or center rumble strips)	Provides both a tactile and an auditory message to the driver about an ongoing road departure condition. They address situations where (1) visibility may be low, (2) drivers may be distracted (e.g., texting), or (3) drivers may be attending to some other task (e.g., sign recognition or general roadway checks), and neglecting lane keeping. Rumble strips are effective since they do not require the driver to be alert and attentive—they can help re-divert an inattentive or sleeping driver's attention back to the driving task and the roadway.
Improved speed management	Provides drivers with more time to make heading corrections and maintain lane position before a lane exceedance turns into a crash.
Markings (e.g., wider longitudinal pavement markings)	Improves the conspicuity/visibility of lane edges and provides drivers with a longer preview time to help them see and respond to lane markings at a greater distance. Especially useful under reduced visibility conditions (e.g., inclement weather, nighttime) or on curves.
Increased lane width (consider context, e.g., rural versus urban)	Allows drivers to maintain lane position with less frequent steering corrections, which correspond to lower levels of driver workload (note that this could encourage higher speeds).
Post-mounted delineators	Improves the conspicuity/visibility of lane edges and provides drivers with a longer preview time to help them see and respond to lane markings and changes in alignment at a greater distance.
Widened shoulders and/or widened "buffer" medians between opposing lanes	Provides drivers more time to correct a lane exceedance before it results in a crash.
TSM&O road weather management strategies (e.g., improved snow preparation) to mitigate weather events (FHWA, 2024)	Improves the conspicuity/visibility of markings and provides drivers with a longer preview time to help them see and respond to them at a greater distance. Especially useful under reduced visibility conditions (e.g., inclement weather, nighttime) or on curves.
Improved roadside hardware and barrier/attenuation systems (e.g., median barriers, cable barriers)	Provides an additional visual cue to delineate the traveled roadway versus the shoulder versus the roadside and can reduce the severity of road departure crashes when they occur.

17% of United States fatalities, up from 14% in 2012 (NCSA, 2023a). In a study examining the efficacy of CMFs for uncontrolled pedestrian crossing treatments, Zegeer et al. (2017) note that there continue to be both (1) safety issues for pedestrians who attempt to cross streets, particularly on high-speed, high-volume, multi-lane roads and (2) a need to better understand the safety effects of some of the more promising treatments on pedestrian crashes.

9.3.3.1 Contributing Factors to Pedestrian Crashes

Driver behavior issues are a key contributor to pedestrian crashes; alcohol was involved in 49% of pedestrian fatalities in 2021 (for the driver and/or the pedestrian) (NCSA, 2023a), and 16% of the fatal 2020 pedestrian crashes involved a driver with a blood alcohol content (BAC) of .08 or higher. Other characteristics of fatal pedestrian crashes are more closely aligned with human factors issues: 84% occurred in urban areas, 75% occurred outside of intersections, and 77% occurred in the dark. While visibility issues seem obvious from the percentage of pedestrian fatalities occurring in the dark, the fatalities occurring in "outside intersections" locations suggest impacts of expectations—drivers are more likely to anticipate pedestrians near intersections.

9.3.3.2 Typical Countermeasures and How They Aid Road Users

Especially in recent years, several technology development efforts and safety evaluations have been conducted to help address crashes and fatalities involving pedestrians. Table 12 highlights

Table 12. Example countermeasures for pedestrian crashes and how they help road users.

Countermeasure	How the Countermeasure Helps Road Users
Advance stop and yield lines	Provides improved visibility of pedestrians for drivers and more time to perceive and react to an unexpected pedestrian incursion by increasing the distance from pedestrians at which drivers are required to stop.
Curb extension/bulb-out	Provides improved visibility and sight distance for pedestrians and vehicles and reduces vehicle speeds, giving drivers more time to react to an unexpected pedestrian incursion. Also, reduces pedestrian exposure by reducing pedestrian crossing times and distances.
Raised median and pedestrian crossing island	Reduces vehicle speeds, providing more time for drivers to perceive and react to an unexpected pedestrian incursion.
Reduce corner radius/crossing distance	Provides improved visibility/sight lines for drivers and reduces turning speeds. Also, reduces pedestrian exposure by reducing pedestrian crossing times and distances.
Pedestrian hybrid beacon or a rectangular rapid flashing beacon	Alerts drivers to the presence of pedestrians in a crosswalk, providing drivers with advance warning and more time to react to the situation.
Right turn on red restrictions	Reduces pedestrian exposure to turning traffic, where line of sight may be blocked or where drivers' attention is divided.
Grade-separated crossings (should only be used when the topography makes them convenient for pedestrians or when the roadway to be crossed is truly inaccessible to pedestrians)	Can eliminate pedestrian exposure to vehicle traffic.
Upgrading traffic signal to include leading pedestrian intervals or protected pedestrian phases	Reduces opportunities for conflicts as pedestrians cross.
Adaptive traffic signal control strategies to address variable demands because of special events, commercial activities or holiday volumes	Traffic signal cycles that can help pedestrians by providing more efficient and effective crossing times.

some of these countermeasures (adapted from Brown et al., 2021) and explains how they help road users by, for example, reducing speeds (thus giving drivers more time to perceive and react to pedestrians) and/or increasing pedestrian visibility and conspicuity.

9.3.4 Bicycle Crashes

Americans are increasingly bicycling to commute, for exercise, or just for fun (NHTSA, n.d.a), and bicyclists are particularly vulnerable to crashes and injuries because they can be less noticeable because of size and a lack of protective structures relative to motor vehicles. In 2021, there were 966 bicyclists (defined as bicyclists and other cyclists on the road, including riders of two-wheel, nonmotorized vehicles, tricycles, and unicycles powered only via pedals) killed in traffic crashes, 95% of which were in single-vehicle crashes (NCSA, 2023b). In addition, there were 41,615 bicyclist injuries in 2021, a 7% increase from 38,886 injuries in 2020 (NCSA, 2023b). Furthermore, bicyclists who were killed in single-vehicle crashes were most likely to be struck by the front of passenger cars and light trucks (NCSA, 2023b).

9.3.4.1 Contributing Factors to Bicycle Crashes

Driver behavior issues are a key contributor to bicycle crashes. Failing to yield the right of way is the highest factor in fatal bike crashes, followed by bicyclists not being visible (NHTSA, n.d.a). In addition, alcohol was involved in 36% of bicyclist fatalities in 2021 (for the driver and/or the bicyclist) and 16% of the fatal 2021 bicyclist crashes involved a driver with a BAC of .08 or higher (NCSA, 2023b). Other characteristics of fatal bicyclist crashes include 85% occurring in urban areas, 29% occurring at intersections, 62% occurring outside of intersections, and 52% occurring in the dark (NCSA, 2023b).

9.3.4.2 Typical Countermeasures and How They Aid Road Users

To help alleviate bicyclist fatalities and injuries, several roadway design improvements can be implemented to benefit all road users. Table 13 highlights some countermeasures that can help minimize conflicts between bicyclists and motor vehicles and improve bicyclist visibility and conspicuity (Brown et al., 2021; National Association of City Transportation Officials [NACTO], 2013; NACTO, 2014; Sando, 2014; Torbic et al., 2014).

9.3.5 Work Zone Crashes

Work zones can impose unique attentional and response demands on road users, including changes in speed limits, awareness of workers in the travel lanes, changing lanes in response

Table 13. Example countermeasures for bicycle crashes and how they help road users.

Countermeasure	How the Countermeasure Helps Road Users
Conventional bicycle lanes	Help support driver expectations for potential bicyclists and where they may be located, and provides improved visibility of bicyclists.
Buffered/separated bicycle lanes	Help support driver expectations for potential bicyclists and where they may be located.
Lane markings/shared lane markings	Help support driver expectations for potential bicyclists and where they may be located, and provides improved visibility of bicyclists.
Two-stage turn queue boxes at intersections	Help support driver expectations for potential bicyclists and where they may be located, provides improved visibility and sight distance of bicyclists, and helps reduce opportunities for conflicts as bicyclists cross the intersection.
Leading bicycle intervals at intersections	Place bicyclists ahead of other vehicles, making them the only travelers in the intersection during the interval. Helps reduce opportunities for conflicts as bicyclists cross the intersection. Provides greater visibility for bicyclists and provides more time for drivers to perceive and react to unexpected bicycle movements.

to lane closures, and making detours around work zone activities. These unique demands have been well-recognized and studied for decades. For example, drivers are generally aware of the conditions associated with work zones and that the presence of traffic control devices (e.g., work-zone-related signs and barrels) provide cues that can help drivers (Kane et al., 1999). The presence of traffic control devices can change driver compliance and responses. A field study measured driver speed selection on highway on-ramps with and without construction-related road signage and found that drivers exhibited reduced speeds when driving in areas with construction-related signage compared to areas without such signage (Tsyganov et al., 2002).

9.3.5.1 Contributing Factors to Work-Zone Crashes

Despite the availability and application of traffic control devices provided by the MUTCD and other sources, many crashes still occur in work zones, and work zone safety is an ongoing issue for researchers, safety practitioners, and policymakers (ARTBA, 2024). While the most frequent crash types in work zones are rear-ended crashes (Garber and Zhao, 2002), fixed-object crashes also occur frequently (Campbell et al., 2012). An analysis of crashes in Kansas highway construction zones showed that fatal work zone crashes in the study region were primarily caused by inattention (53% of fatal crashes), speeding (25%), and disregarding traffic control (21%) (Li and Bai, 2008).

9.3.5.2 Typical Countermeasures and How They Aid Road Users

Since rear-end collisions are the predominant type of work zone crash, engineers and other practitioners have focused on providing warnings in advance of work zones to support driver expectations for reduced speeds and increased vigilance, as well as measures for improving speed control and setting appropriate work zone speed limits. The general purpose of work zone design elements is to provide warning, delineation, and channelization information to help road users in advance of and through a work zone. Table 14 highlights some of these countermeasures and explains how they help road users by, for example, providing advance information to enhance expectations and reduce speeds (thus giving drivers more time to perceive and react to conditions).

Table 14. Example countermeasures for work zone crashes and how they help road users (adapted from: Antonucci et al., 2005; Campbell et al., 2012).

Countermeasure	How the Countermeasure Helps Road Users
Portable changeable message signs	Provide advance warning of an upcoming work zone and/or revisions to normal speeds or vehicle routes; help support driver expectations for upcoming deviations from normal driving conditions
Arrow boards	Provide additional warning and directional information to inform drivers of upcoming lane closures; help support driver expectations for upcoming deviations from normal driving conditions
Speed warning systems	Communicate speeds downstream on variable message signs to inform drivers that they may soon need to slow down or stop; enhance expectations about speed changes and give drivers more time to react to conditions downstream
Changes to lane widths and number of available lanes	Support lower speeds (mean vehicle speed reductions are correlated with the number of open lanes and lane widths)
511 services	Support expectations and trip planning activities by providing information about closures, delays, and suggested detour routes
Variable speed limit systems	Adjust work zone speeds based on time-of-day, weather, traffic volumes or other variables—can match speeds to conditions in work zones and improve available response times for all road users

9.3.6 Intersection Crashes

Motor vehicle crashes at intersections are common since vehicle paths naturally conflict at intersections as roads cross one another or as individual vehicles turn left or right against or into oncoming vehicles. Bikes and pedestrians also use intersections and are especially vulnerable at locations where their paths intersect with one another and with larger, faster-moving vehicles. According to 2008 data obtained through the FARS and the National Automotive Sampling System-General Estimates System (NASS-GES), approximately 40% of the estimated 5,811,000 crashes that occurred in the United States occurred at intersections or were intersection-related crashes (NHTSA, 2008b).

9.3.6.1 Contributory Factors to Intersection Crashes

The NHTSA examined the contributing factors associated with intersection-related crashes as part of the NMVCCS. NMVCCS data were collected from January 2005 to December 2007 and include on-scene information on the conditions and associated factors leading up to a crash (Choi, 2010). Thirty-six percent (787,236) of the total (2,188,969) NMVCCS crashes were intersection-related, and about 96% of the intersection-related crashes had critical reasons attributed to drivers (Choi, 2010). Of those crashes where the critical reason was attributed to the driver, 55% were associated with recognition errors such as inadequate surveillance, internal distractions, or inattention; 29% were attributed to decision errors such as false assumption of other's actions or misjudgment of gap or other's speed (Choi, 2010).

9.3.6.2 Typical Countermeasures and How They Help

For both signalized and unsignalized intersections, the predominant crash types are angle, rear-end, pedestrian, and bicyclist crashes. Accordingly, practitioners have focused on countermeasures that improve visibility, provide road users with more time to make decisions and react, and support complex crossing movements that can intersect with other road users' movements. Table 15 highlights some of these countermeasures and explains how they help road users.

Table 15. Example countermeasures for intersection crashes and how they help road users (adapted from: Antonucci et al., 2005; Campbell et al., 2012).

Countermeasure	How the Countermeasure Helps Road Users
Adding a "Signal Ahead" warning sign	Provides advance warning of an upcoming sign, especially in situations where sight distance to a signal head may not be adequate for unfamiliar drivers who do not expect the traffic signal to stop comfortably on a red light
Adding traffic signal backplates or increasing signal head size	Improves conspicuity and visibility of the traffic signals
Adding a protected left-turn phase to the traffic signal	Reduces surveillance requirements and workload on turning drivers by reducing the need to assess gaps (i.e., to assess speed and distance of oncoming vehicles) when turning
Eliminating parking ahead of an intersection	Improves driver sight distance and visibility of pedestrians and bicyclists as drivers approach an unsignalized intersection
Installing turn lanes, increasing the length of an existing left-turn lane, or restricting movements to right-in/right-out at unsignalized intersections	Where crashes seem to be associated with driveways or other access points, these can reduce rear-end crashes associated with unexpected left turns and provide drivers with more time to prepare for the turn. Movement restrictions reduce workload and associated surveillance requirements for turning drivers and for adjacent vehicles
Adding safe turning lanes in the form of roundabouts	Can reduce conflict points and workload at an intersection and reduce or mitigate crashes

Key Concepts

1. Effective countermeasures decrease the demands placed on the road user and/or augment the road user's capabilities in some fashion.
2. Countermeasures should be selected in a manner that links their features and benefits to the underlying contributing crash factors and human factors issues/aberrant driver behavior issues observed within the crash data or the facility itself.
3. Final countermeasure selection should include trade-offs between key variables, including countermeasure efficacy, specific safety benefits, unanticipated outcomes, and feasibility (e.g., time and cost).

CHAPTER 10

Decision Trees to Support Countermeasure Selection

10.1 Background

This chapter provides a series of decision trees to help practitioners select countermeasures to address target crash types and facility types. Decision trees provide a visual framework for decision-making. Practitioners can select from a series of decision trees that lead them through diagnostic questions to help identify countermeasures that could potentially address crash-contributing factors associated with the crash pattern of interest. Selecting countermeasures for potential implementation, matched to underlying contributing factors to target crash types, is expected to reduce crashes to the greatest extent possible.

The decision trees presented here are based on the logic of the diagnostic scenarios incorporated in the Safety Analyst software (Harwood et al., 2010), a former AASHTOWare product that implemented and automated the six main steps of the roadway safety management process outlined in HSM Part B. As part of the third step in the roadway safety management process, the software led an engineer/analyst through a series of questions to identify crash-contributing factors related to particular crash types at a site and identify potential countermeasures to remedy the contributing factors associated with the crash type of interest. The primary result of reviewing and answering the diagnostic questions is a list of potential countermeasures for further consideration in the economic appraisal and project prioritization process to select those countermeasures for implementation that are most cost-effective.

In addition to the logic of diagnostic scenarios incorporated in the Safety Analyst software, the decision trees presented here have been adapted to include additional diagnostic questions and reflect additional countermeasure information gathered from sources including the following:

- PEDSAFE: Pedestrian Safety Guide and Countermeasure Selection System (FHWA, n.d.c)
- BIKESAFE: Bicycle Safety Guide and Countermeasure Selection System (FHWA, n.d.a)
- United States Road Assessment Program (usRAP) (Roadway Safety Foundation, 2024b)
- The *HFG for Road Systems: Fourth Edition* (upcoming)
- CMF Clearinghouse (FHWA, n.d.b)
- *Field Guide for Selecting Countermeasures at Uncontrolled Pedestrian Crossing Locations* (Blackburn et al., 2018)

10.2 Crash Types

Decision trees have been developed to address common crash types and countermeasures included in many state SHSPs and for which states use HSIP funds. According to the *HSIP 2019 National Summary Report* (Albee and Gross, 2021), states use HSIP funds to address several predominant infrastructure-related crash types, including roadway departure, intersection, and pedestrian crashes. Current data on HSIP activities and success stories in the United States are compiled and published by the FHWA (FHWA, 2023a). Figure 20 shows the top 11 state safety programs administered under HSIP. Over half of the states have roadway departure (26 states) and intersection (26 states) safety programs, while 20 states have pedestrian safety programs, and agencies are spending their HSIP funds on projects consistent with their top programs. Figure 21 presents the number of HSIP projects categorized by common SHSP emphasis areas. Approximately 35% of the HSIP projects were categorized as intersections, 32% were categorized as roadway departures, and 8% were categorized as pedestrians.

Thus, the decision trees included here are consistent with the common crash types and types of safety projects being addressed by states. The decision trees also address pedestrian and bicycle crashes as these are of high interest to agencies across the United States, as evidenced by the U.S. DOT announcing new guidance to improve the safety of VRUs (FHWA, 2022b).

Table 16 presents a roadmap for the decision trees to help guide countermeasure selection. Decision trees address common crash types that occur along rural and urban roadway segments and intersections, including the following:

- Rural two-lane roadway segments
- Rural multilane undivided roadway segments
- Rural multilane divided roadway segments
- Urban two-lane roadway segments
- Urban multilane undivided roadway segments
- Urban multilane divided roadway segments
- Rural and urban signalized intersections
- Rural and urban unsignalized intersections

The crash types are further categorized according to common crash contributing factors. Through the diagnostic process, practitioners should get a sense of the factors contributing to the crash pattern of interest. Then, by reviewing the respective decision trees, following the logic, and responding to the questions, practitioners will be able to identify a list of potential countermeasures for further consideration in the economic appraisal and project prioritization process. When selecting countermeasures for potential implementation, practitioners should also consider building redundancy into the system consistent with a Safe System.

As shown in Table 16, some of the crash types and contributing factors are common across the various roadway contexts (i.e., site types). As such, some of the diagnostic scenarios apply

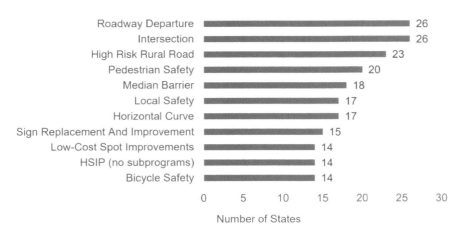

*Figure 20.   **Number of state safety programs (Source: Albee and Gross, 2021).***

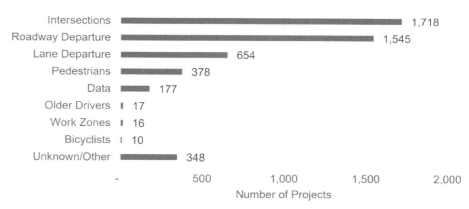

Figure 21. Number of HSIP projects by SHSP emphasis areas (Source: Albee and Gross, 2021).

to more than one context (i.e., site type). In some situations, though, the same diagnostic questions may be asked, but the potential countermeasures may differ given the context. Table 17 can be used in conjunction with several decision trees for pedestrian and bicycle crashes, including the decision trees in Figures 62, 63, 71, 72, 76, 77, and 101, as these decision trees refer to Table 17 for additional guidance related to countermeasures for uncontrolled crossing locations.

As users of this toolbox work through the logic of these decision trees to identify a list of potential countermeasures for further consideration in the economic appraisal and project prioritization process, users should exercise engineering judgment and identify trade-offs to assess the applicability of the potential countermeasures to the individual site or sites of interest. The potential countermeasures identified through the diagnostic scenarios may not apply to the individual site or sites of interest. Also, the list of potential countermeasures identified is not necessarily exhaustive. That is, users should also consider the potential implementation of additional countermeasures not identified through the diagnostic scenarios. These decision trees serve to address general conditions and the potential countermeasures identified through the diagnostic scenarios should not be considered as the only countermeasures applicable to remedy the target crash type at the site or sites of interest.

Additionally, the list of potential countermeasures that may be identified using the logic of a given decision tree is not presented in any type of prioritized order for implementation. For example, the first diagnostic question of Figure 26 in reference to rural two-lane segments, roadway departure crashes, and road surface conditions is, "Does the pavement surface near curves where crashes were recorded show signs of deterioration, ponding, polishing, or icing?" If the user responds "Yes," the potential countermeasures for implementation are presented for consideration as follows:

- Improve pavement friction
- Maintain or improve the surface of lanes
- Improve drainage patterns or structures
- Apply preventative salting or chemical anti-icing
- Install high-friction surface treatment

The order of countermeasures presented from top to bottom in the decision tree figures is not intended to signify any type of prioritization for countermeasure selection or implementation. Priority for selection and implementation is to be based on the applicability of the countermeasure to remedy the crash type of interest at the given site, the cost effectiveness of the implementation of the countermeasure, and other factors, such as trade-offs in safety and

Table 16. Decision trees to support countermeasure selection.

Crash Type	Type of Segment and Contributing Factor	Figure No.	Page No.
Rural Two-Lane Segments			
Roadway departure crashes (single-vehicle run-off-road)	Driver inattention / impairment	22	90
	Roadside design	23	92
	Speed / curvature / guidance	24	95
	Roadway surface condition / superelevation	25	97
	Roadway surface condition / drainage	26	98
Roadway departure crashes (head-on / sideswipe, opposite direction)	Driver inattention / impairment	27	100
	Roadside design	28	102
	Overtaking	29	103
	Speed / curvature / guidance	30	105
	Roadway surface condition / superelevation	25	97
	Roadway surface condition / drainage	26	98
Rear-end crashes	Driveways / accesses	31	106
	Roadway surface condition / drainage	26	98
Pedestrian crashes	Dart-dash / midblock / along the road	32	108
Bicycle crashes	Bicyclist rode out midblock / motorist turned into path of bicyclist / bicyclist turned into path / overtaking	33	110
Rural Multilane Undivided Segments			
Roadway departure crashes (single-vehicle run-off-road)	Driver inattention / impairment	34	112
	Roadside design	35	114
	Speed / curvature / guidance	36	117
	Roadway surface condition / superelevation	37	119
	Roadway surface condition / drainage	38	120
Roadway departure crashes (head-on / sideswipe, opposite direction)	Driver inattention / impairment	39	122
	Roadside design	40	123
	Speed / curvature / guidance	41	125
	Roadway surface condition / superelevation	37	119
	Roadway surface condition / drainage	38	120
Rear-end crash	Driveways / accesses	42	126
	Roadway surface condition / drainage	38	120
Pedestrian crashes	Dart-dash / midblock / along the road	43	128
Bicycle crashes	Bicyclist rode out midblock / motorist turned into path of bicyclist / bicyclist turned into path / overtaking	44	130
Rural Multilane Divided Segments			
Roadway departure crashes (single-vehicle run-off-road)	Driver inattention / impairment	45	132
	Roadside design	46	134
	Speed / curvature / guidance	47	137
	Roadway surface condition / superelevation	48	139
	Roadway surface condition / drainage	49	140
Roadway departure crashes (head-on / sideswipe, opposite direction)	Driver inattention / impairment	50	141
	Median design	51	142
	Speed / curvature / guidance	52	143
Rear-end crash	Driveways / accesses	53	145
	Roadway surface condition / drainage	49	140
Pedestrian crashes	Dart-dash / midblock / along the road	54	147
Bicycle crashes	Bicyclist rode out midblock / motorist turned into path of bicyclist / bicyclist turned into path / overtaking	55	149

Table 16.   (Continued).

Crash Type	Type of Segment and Contributing Factor	Figure No.	Page No.
Urban Two-lane Segments			
Roadway departure crashes (single-vehicle run-off-road)	Roadside design	56	151
	Speed / curvature / guidance	57	153
	Roadway surface condition / drainage	58	154
Roadway departure crashes (head-on / sideswipe, opposite direction)	Roadway surface condition / drainage	58	154
	Overtaking	59	156
	Driver inattention / impairment	60	157
Rear-end crashes	Roadway surface condition / drainage	58	154
	Driveways / accesses	61	158
Angle crashes	Driveways / accesses	61	158
Pedestrian crashes	Dart-dash / midblock / along the road	62	160
Bicycle crashes	Bicyclist rode out midblock / motorist turned into path of bicyclist / bicyclist turned into path / overtaking	63	162
Urban Multilane Undivided Segments			
Roadway departure crashes (single-vehicle run-off-road)	Roadside design	64	164
	Speed / curvature / guidance	65	165
	Roadway surface condition / drainage	66	166
Roadway departure crashes (head-on / sideswipe, opposite direction)	Roadway surface condition / drainage	66	166
	Driver inattention / impairment	67	168
	Speed / curvature / guidance	68	169
Sideswipe, same direction crashes	Speed / curvature / guidance	69	170
	Driveways / accesses	70	171
Rear-end crashes	Driveways / accesses	70	171
Angle crashes	Driveways / accesses	70	171
Pedestrian crashes	Dart-dash / midblock / along the road	71	173
Bicycle crashes	Bicyclist rode out midblock / motorist turned into path of bicyclist / bicyclist turned into path / overtaking	72	175
Urban Multilane Divided Segments			
Roadway departure crashes (single-vehicle run-off-road)	Roadway surface condition / drainage	73	177
	Speed / curvature / guidance	74	179
Sideswipe, same direction crashes	Roadway surface condition / drainage	73	177
	Speed / curvature / guidance	74	179
	Driveways / accesses	75	180
Rear-end crashes	Roadway surface condition / drainage	73	177
	Driveways / accesses	75	180
Angle crashes	Driveways / accesses	75	180
Pedestrian crashes	Dart-dash / midblock / along the road	76	182
Bicycle crashes	Bicyclist rode out midblock / motorist turned into path of bicyclist / bicyclist turned into path / overtaking	77	184
Rural and Urban Signalized Intersections			
Angle crashes	Signal visibility	78	187
	Signal timing / capacity	79	189
	Speed	80	190
	Pavement friction	81	191
	Sight distance	82	193
	Driver running red light	83	194
	Driver gap acceptance	84	195
	Driver inattention and/or lack of road messages	85	196
	Driveways / accesses	86	198

(continued on next page)

Table 16. (Continued).

Crash Type	Type of Segment and Contributing Factor	Figure No.	Page No.
Rear-end crashes	Signal visibility	78	187
	Signal timing / capacity	87	200
	Speed	88	202
	Pavement friction	81	191
	Sight distance (for turns)	89	203
	Driver gap acceptance	84	195
	Guidance / road messages	90	204
	Driveways / accesses	86	198
	Unexpected stops on approach	91	205
Pedestrian crashes	Dash-dart / multiple threat / turning vehicle / through vehicle	92	206
Bicycle crashes	Motorist failed to yield / bicyclist failed to yield / turning vehicle	93	209
Rural and Urban Unsignalized Intersections			
Angle crashes / rear-end crashes	Stop sign visibility	94	211
	Sight distance	95	213
	Speed	96	215
	Pavement friction	97	216
	Driver gap acceptance	98	218
	Driver inattention and/or lack of road messages	99	220
	Driveways / accesses	100	222
Pedestrian crashes	Dash-dart / multiple threat / turning vehicle / through vehicle	101	224
Bicycle crashes	Motorist failed to yield / bicyclist failed to yield / turning vehicle	102	226

Table 17. Suggested countermeasures for uncontrolled crossing locations (Source: Blackburn et al., 2018).

Roadway Configuration	Speed Limit								
	Vehicle AADT <9,000			Vehicle AADT 9,000–15,000			Vehicle AADT >15,000		
	≤30 mph	35 mph	≥40 mph	≤30 mph	35 mph	≥40 mph	≤30 mph	35 mph	≥40 mph
2 lanes*	**1** 2 3 4 5 6	**1** **3** 5 6 7	**1** **3** 5 6 **7**	**1** 3 4 5 6	**1** **3** 5 6 7	**1** **3** 5 6 **7**	**1** 3 4 5 6 7	**1** **3** 5 6 7	**1** **3** 5 6 **7**
3 lanes with raised median*	**1** 2 3 4 5	**1** **3** 5 7	**1** **3** 5 **7**	**1** 3 4 5 7	**1** **3** 5 **7**	**1** **3** 5 **7**	**1** **3** 4 5 7	**1** **3** 5 **7**	**1** **3** 5 **7**
3 lanes w/o raised median†	**1** 2 3 4 5 6 7	**1** **3** 5 6 7	**1** **3** 5 6 **7**	**1** 3 4 5 6 7	**1** **3** 5 6 **7**	**1** **3** 5 6 **7**	**1** **3** 4 5 6 7	**1** **3** 5 6 **7**	**1** **3** 5 6 **7**
4+ lanes with raised median‡	**1** **3** 5	**1** **3** 5	**1** **3** 5 7	**1** **3** 5	**1** **3** 5 7	**1** **3** 5 **7**	**1** **3** 5	**1** **3** 5 **7**	**1** **3** 5 **7**
4+ lanes w/o raised median‡	**1** **3** 5 6 7 8	**1** **3** 5 **6** 7 8	**1** **3** 5 **6** **7** 8	**1** **3** 5 **6** 7 8	**1** **3** 5 **6** **7** 8	**1** **3** 5 **6** **7** 8	**1** **3** 5 **6** **7** 8	**1** **3** 5 **6** **7** 8	**1** **3** 5 **6** **7** 8

*One lane in each direction   †One lane in each direction with two-way left-turn lane   ‡Two or more lanes in each direction

Given the set of conditions in a cell,

● Signifies that the countermeasure should always be considered, but not mandated or required, based upon engineering judgment at a marked uncontrolled crossing location.

\# Signifies that the countermeasure is a candidate treatment at a marked uncontrolled crossing location.

The absence of a number signifies that the countermeasure is generally not an appropriate treatment, but exceptions may be considered following engineering judgment.

1 High-visibility crosswalk markings, parking restriction on crosswalk approach, adequate nighttime lighting levels
2 Raised crosswalk
3 Advance Yield Here To (Stop Here For) Pedestrians sign and yield (stop) line
4 In-Street Pedestrian Crossing sign
5 Curb extension
6 Pedestrian refuge island
7 Pedestrian Hybrid Beacon
8 Road Diet

This table was developed using information from: Zeegeer, C. V., Stewart, J. R., Huang, H. H., Lagerwey, P. A., Feaganes, J., & Campbell, B. J. (2005). Safety effects of marked versus unmarked crosswalks at uncontrolled locations: Final report and recommended guidelines (No. FHWA-HRT-04-100); Manual on Uniform Traffic Control Devices, 2009 Edition, Chapter 4F. Pedestrian Hybrid Beacons; the Crash Modification Factors (CMF) Clearinghouse website (http://www.cmfclearinghouse.org/); and the Pedestrian Safety Guide and Countermeasure Selection System (PEDSAFE) website (http://www.pedbikesafe.org/PEDSAFE/).

mobility between all road users. The user may want to give a countermeasure greater consideration for implementation if (1) the countermeasure was identified for implementation more than once in response to different diagnostic questions or (2) when the same countermeasure was identified for potential implementation in response to different combinations of contexts, crash types, and contributing factors. Even in these situations, the economic appraisal and project prioritization process, following countermeasure selection, will provide additional details to inform decisions regarding prioritization for implementation based on economic performance measures.

Several of the decision trees have one or two questions related to speed. However, in most of the diagnostic scenarios, reducing speeds either along the roadway segment or the approach to the intersection may likely reduce crash frequencies and severities. Thus, as a general rule of thumb, users should consider various speed management techniques, either through the implementation of traffic control devices, changes to the roadway geometrics, and installation of traffic calming treatments and gateway treatments to reduce the frequency and severity of the target crashes. In general, if you cannot reduce speeds, you should separate road users in space. Implementation of speed management techniques to reduce operating speeds is consistent with the Safe System Approach to reduce system kinetic energy.

Finally, countermeasure selection should include trade-offs between key variables, including safety considerations for all road users, redundancy in the system, countermeasure efficacy, specific safety benefits, unanticipated outcomes, and feasibility (e.g., time and cost). In particular, users should also identify trade-offs in safety and mobility between motorists, pedestrians, and bicyclists that may arise from potential countermeasures, including unintended consequences to other road users. For example, potential countermeasures may be identified to reduce the crash frequency of certain types of multiple-vehicle crashes (e.g., rear-end or angle); but before selecting a countermeasure for further consideration in the economic appraisal and project prioritization process, the user should also consider potential trade-offs for pedestrians or bicyclists. A countermeasure expected to reduce rear-end or angle crashes at a site may also be expected to increase the exposure of pedestrians and bicyclists to motor vehicle traffic and, in turn, may increase the frequency of pedestrian and bicycle crashes. As users are identifying countermeasures for further consideration in the economic appraisal and project prioritization process and their potential applicability at an individual site or sites, users are to make informed decisions considering the trade-offs in safety and mobility between motorists, pedestrians, and bicyclists that may arise from potential countermeasures.

10.3 Rural Two-lane Segments

Figure 22 to Figure 33 present the decision trees for rural two-lane segments.

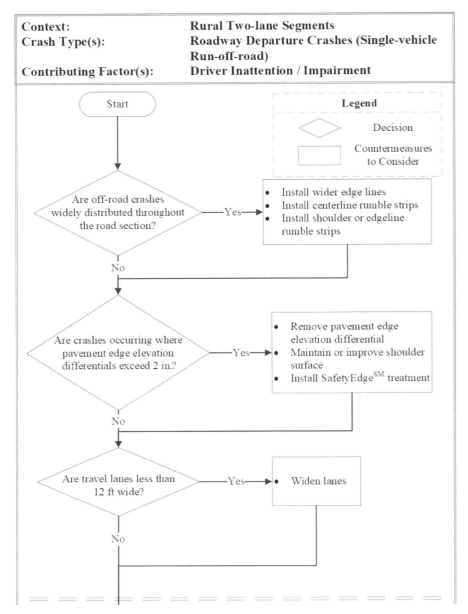

Figure 22. Rural two-lane segments; roadway departure crashes (single-vehicle run-off-road); driver inattention/impairment (Source for information on supplementing standard centerline markings: Brewer and Bedsole, 2015; Albin et al., 2016).

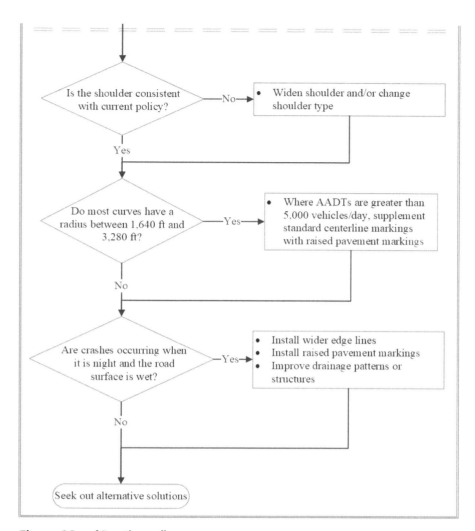

Figure 22. (Continued).

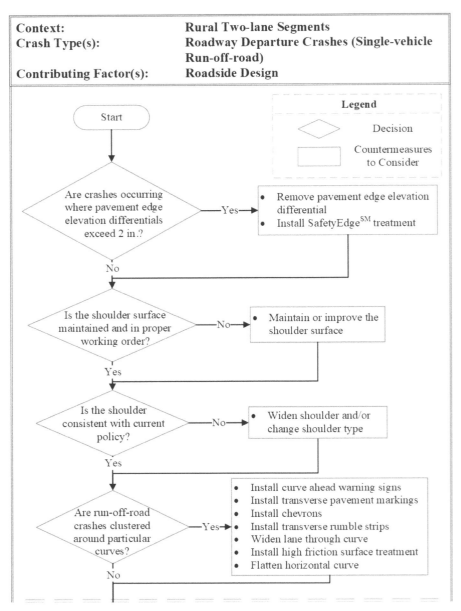

Context:	Rural Two-lane Segments
Crash Type(s):	Roadway Departure Crashes (Single-vehicle Run-off-road)
Contributing Factor(s):	Roadside Design

Figure 23.   Rural two-lane segments; roadway departure crashes (single-vehicle run-off-road); roadside design.

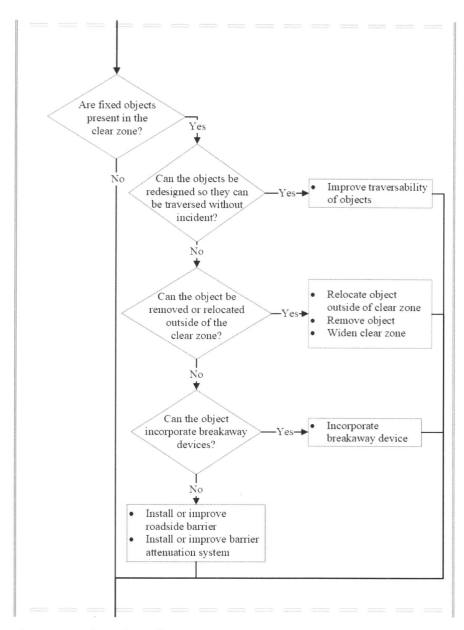

Figure 23.   (Continued).

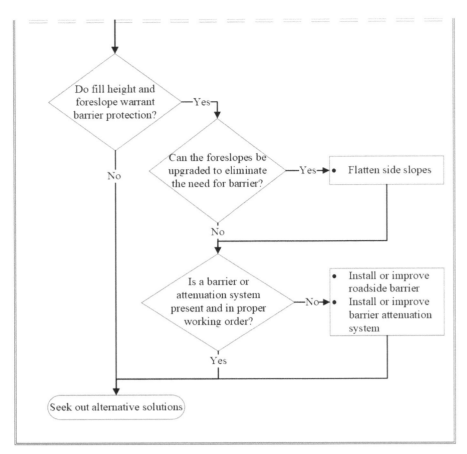

Figure 23. *(Continued)*.

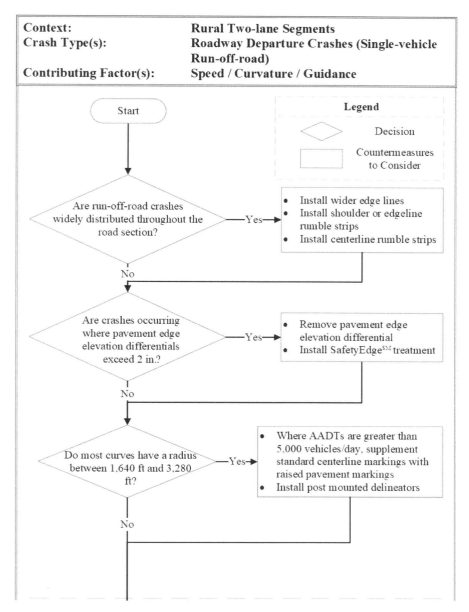

Figure 24. Rural two-lane segments; roadway departure crashes (single-vehicle run-off-road); speed/curvature/guidance (Source for information on supplementing standard centerline markings: Brewer and Bedsole, 2015; Albin et al., 2016).

(continued on next page)

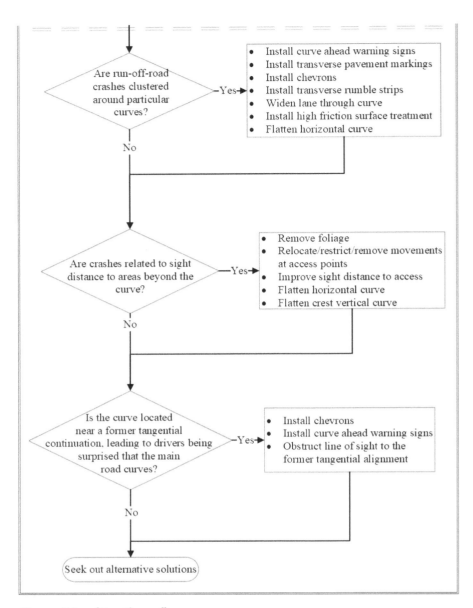

Figure 24. *(Continued).*

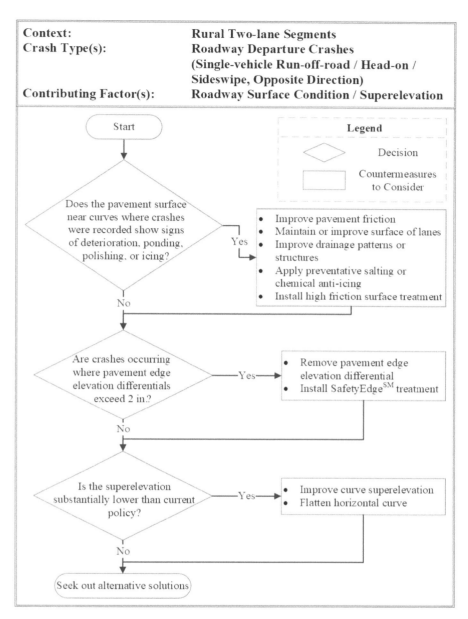

Figure 25. Rural two-lane segments; roadway departure crashes (single-vehicle run-off-road/head-on/sideswipe, opposite direction); roadway surface condition/superelevation.

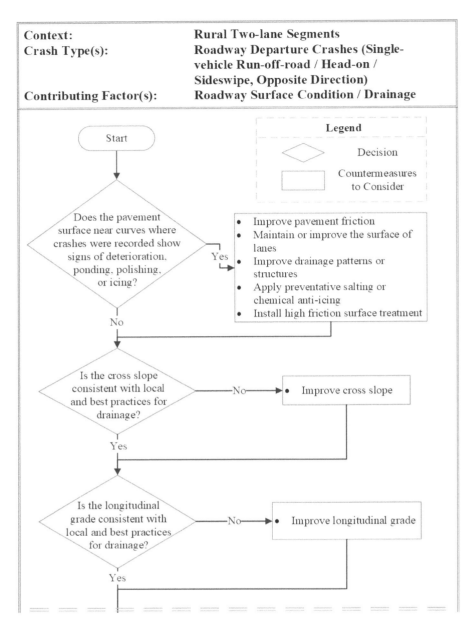

Figure 26.   Rural two-lane segments; roadway departure crashes (single-vehicle run-off-road/head-on/sideswipe, opposite direction), roadway surface condition/drainage.

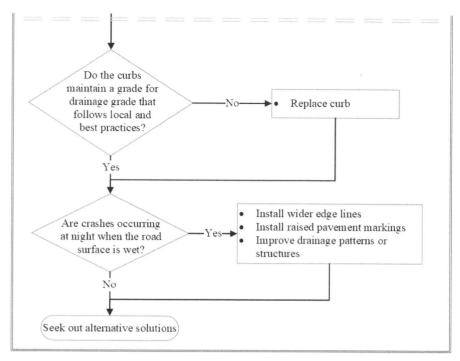

Figure 26.   (Continued).

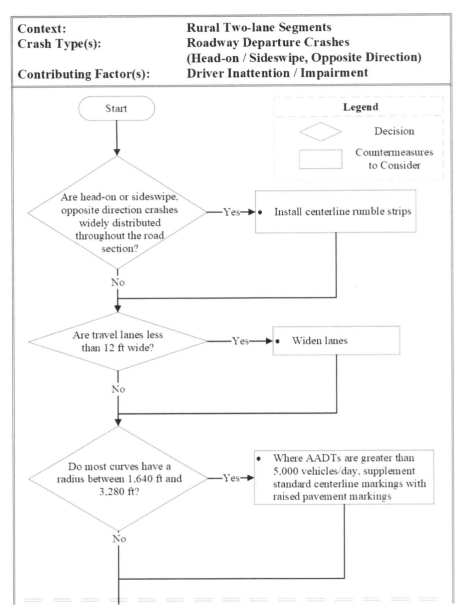

Figure 27. Rural two-lane segments; roadway departure crashes (head-on/sideswipe, opposite direction); driver inattention/impairment (Source for information on supplementing standard centerline markings: Brewer and Bedsole, 2015; Albin et al., 2016).

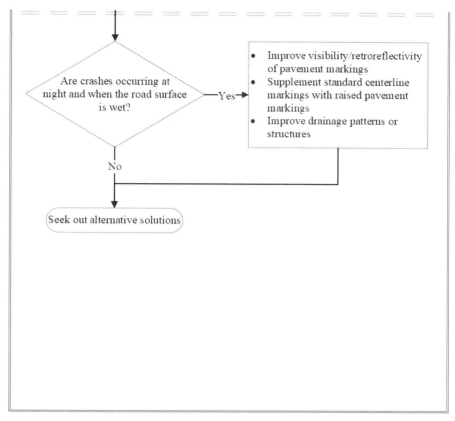

Figure 27. *(Continued).*

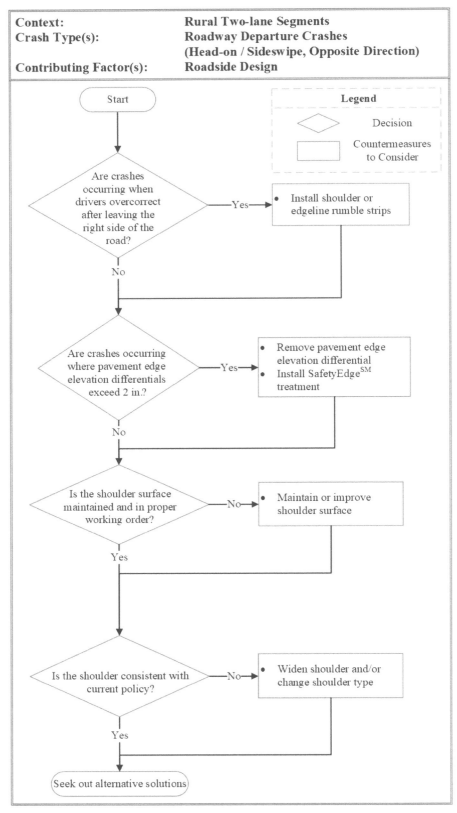

Figure 28.   Rural two-lane segments; roadway departure crashes (head-on/sideswipe, opposite direction); roadside design.

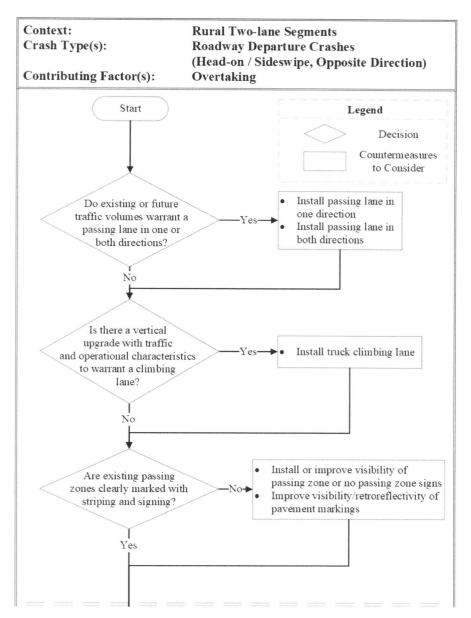

Context: **Rural Two-lane Segments**
Crash Type(s):   **Roadway Departure Crashes**
                           (Head-on / Sideswipe, Opposite Direction)
Contributing Factor(s):   **Overtaking**

Figure 29. Rural two-lane segments; roadway departure crashes (head-on/sideswipe, opposite direction); overtaking.

(continued on next page)

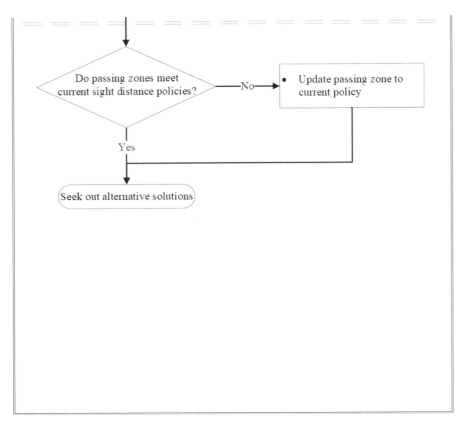

Figure 29.   (Continued).

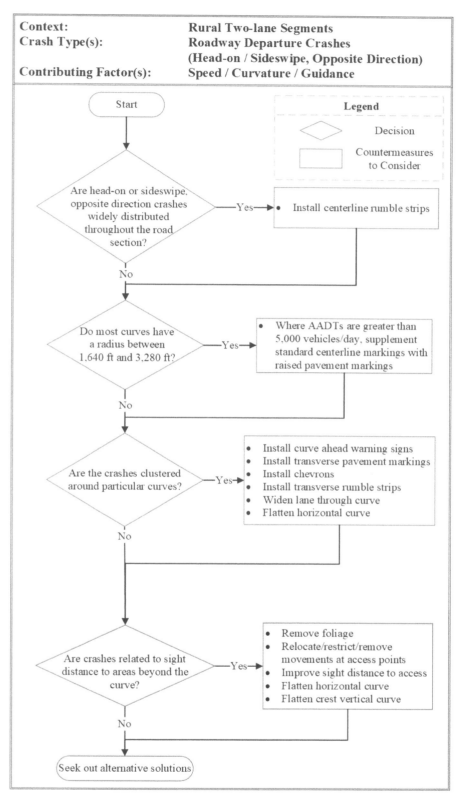

*Figure 30.   Rural two-lane segments; roadway departure crashes
(head-on/sideswipe, opposite direction); speed/curvature/guidance
(Source for information on supplementing standard centerline
markings: Brewer and Bedsole, 2015; Albin et al., 2016).*

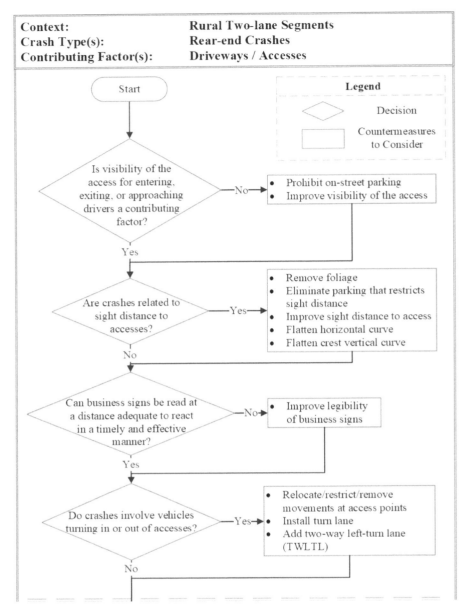

Figure 31.   Rural two-lane segments; rear-end crashes; driveways/ accesses.

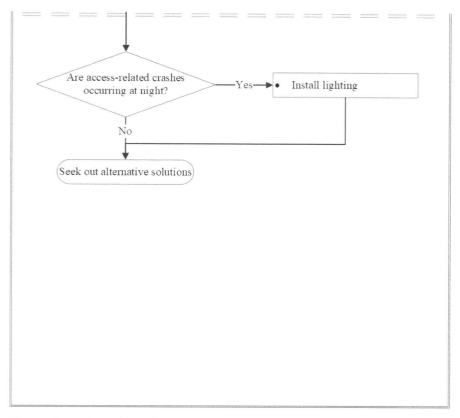

Figure 31.   (Continued).

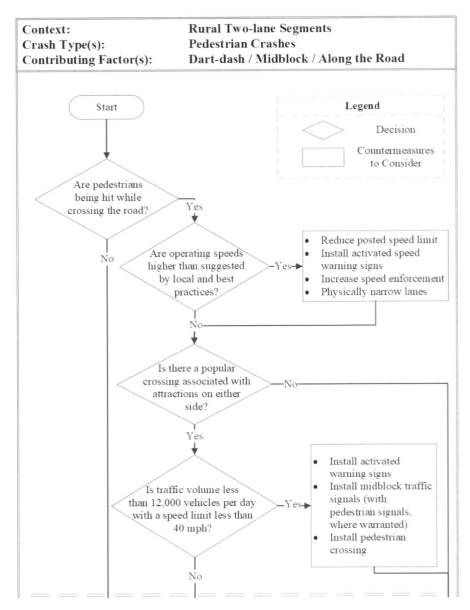

Figure 32.   Rural two-lane segments; pedestrian crashes; dart-dash/ midblock/along the road.

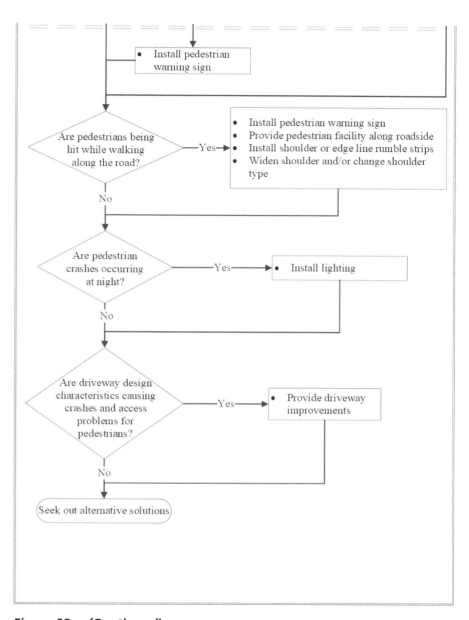

Figure 32.   (Continued).

Context: Rural Two-lane Segments
Crash Type(s): Bicycle Crashes
Contributing Factor(s): Bicyclist Rode out Midblock / Motorist Turned into Path of Bicyclist / Bicyclist Turned into Path / Overtaking

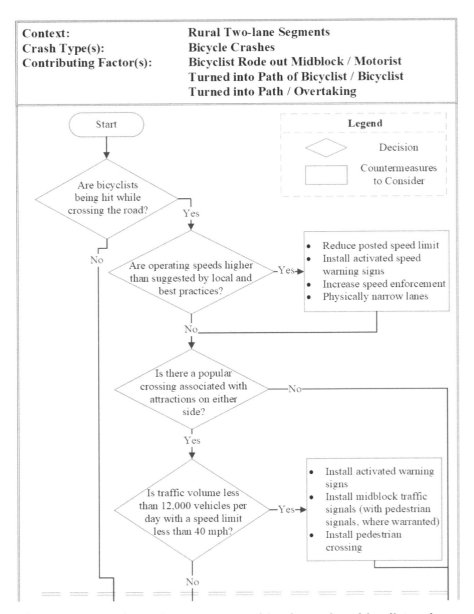

Figure 33. Rural two-lane segments; bicycle crashes; bicyclist rode out midblock/motorist turned into path of bicyclist/bicyclist turned into path/overtaking.

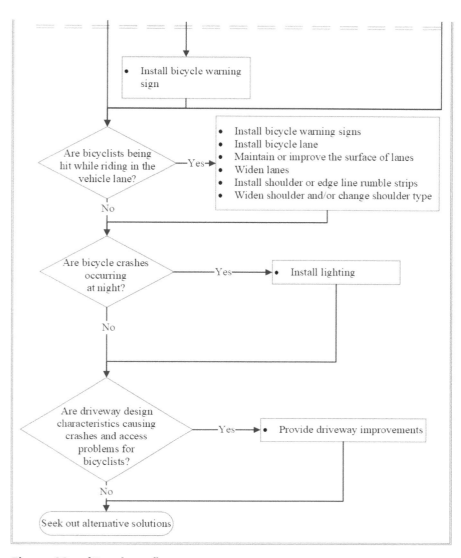

Figure 33. (Continued).

10.4 Rural Multilane Undivided Segments

Figures 34 to 44 present the decision trees for rural multilane undivided segments.

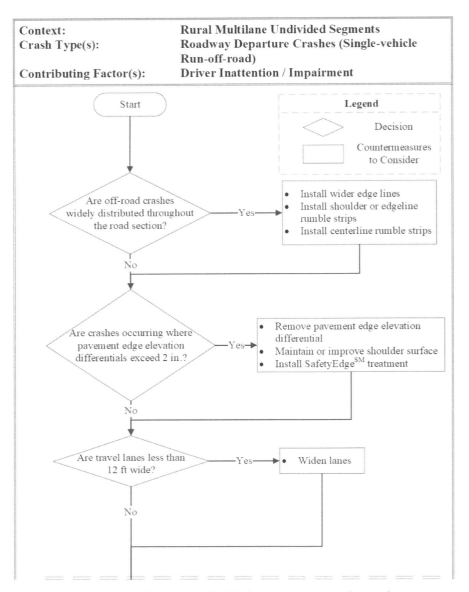

Figure 34.   Rural multilane undivided segments; roadway departure crashes (single-vehicle run-off-road); driver inattention/impairment (Source for information on supplementing standard centerline markings: Brewer and Bedsole, 2015; Albin et al., 2016).

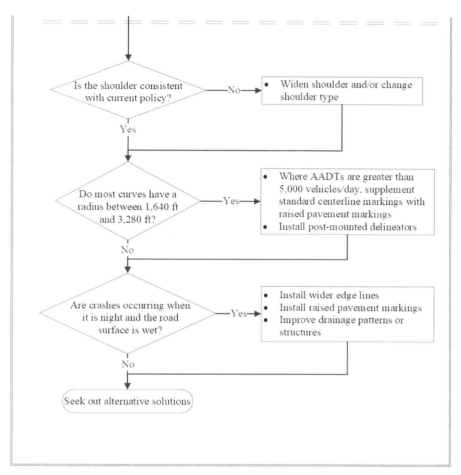

Figure 34.   (Continued).

Context:	Rural Multilane Undivided Segments
Crash Type(s):	Roadway Departure Crashes (Single-vehicle Run-off-road)
Contributing Factor(s):	Roadside Design

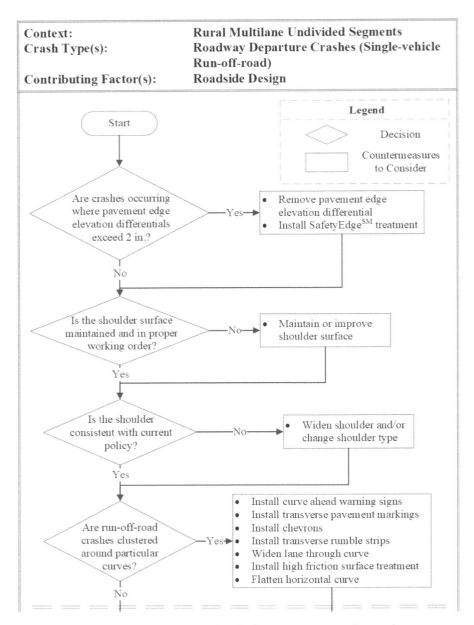

Figure 35. Rural multilane undivided segments; roadway departure crashes (single-vehicle run-off-road); roadside design.

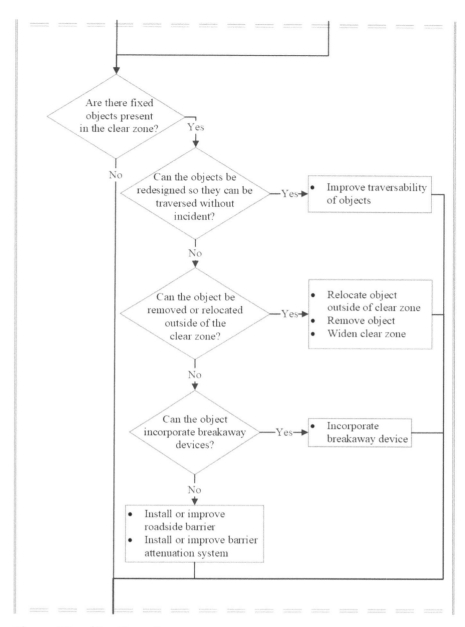

Figure 35.   (Continued).

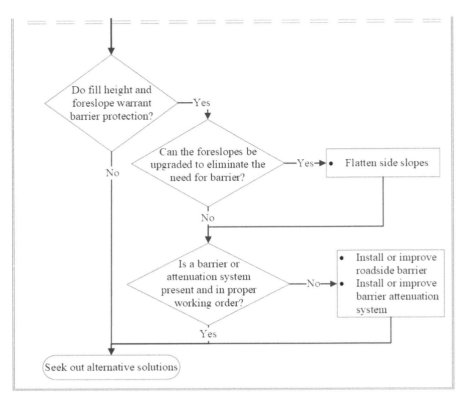

Figure 35. (Continued).

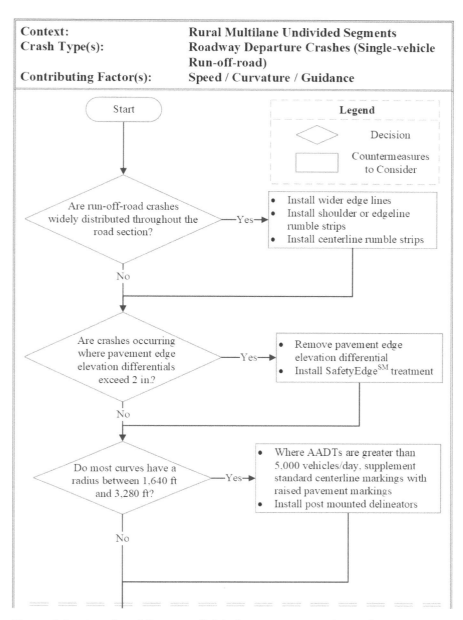

Figure 36.   Rural multilane undivided segments; roadway departure crashes (single-vehicle run-off-road); speed/curvature/guidance (Source for information on supplementing standard centerline markings: Brewer and Bedsole, 2015; Albin et al., 2016).

(continued on next page)

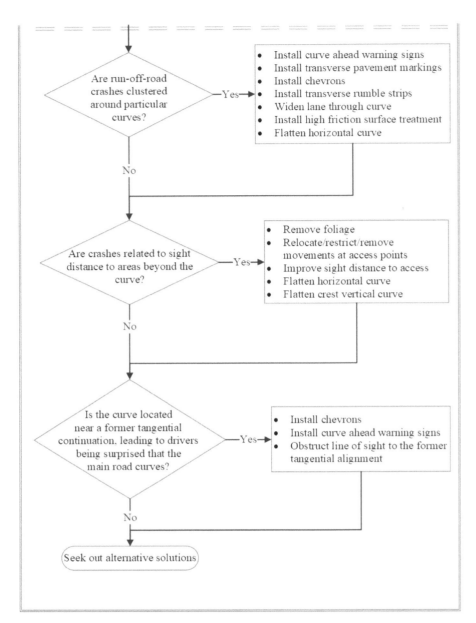

Figure 36.   (Continued).

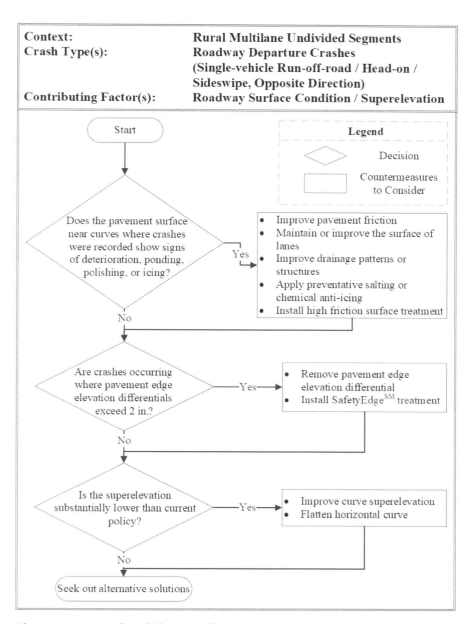

Figure 37.   Rural multilane undivided segments: roadway departure crashes (single-vehicle run-off-road/head-on/sideswipe, opposite direction); roadway surface condition/superelevation.

Context:	**Rural Multilane Undivided Segments**
Crash Type(s):	**Roadway Departure Crashes (Single-vehicle Run-off-road / Head-on / Sideswipe, Opposite Direction), Rear-end Crashes**
Contributing Factor(s):	**Roadway Surface Condition / Drainage**

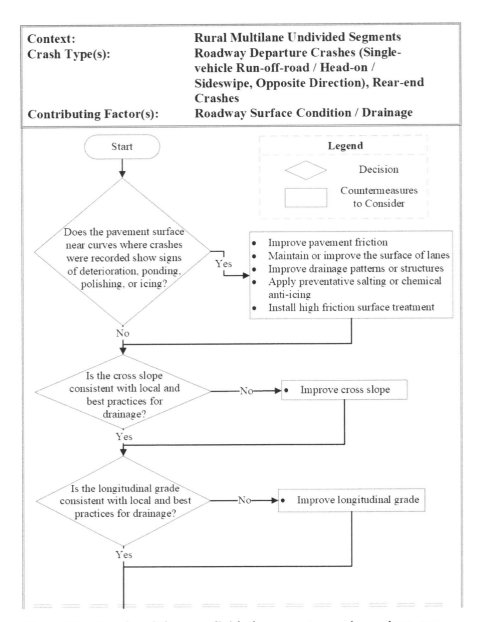

Figure 38.   Rural multilane undivided segments; roadway departure crashes (single-vehicle run-off-road/head-on/rear-end/sideswipe, opposite direction); rear-end crashes; roadway surface condition/drainage.

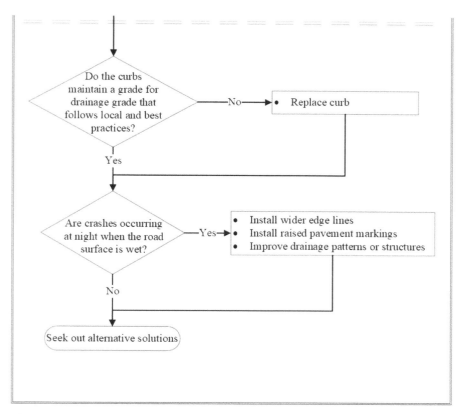

Figure 38. (Continued).

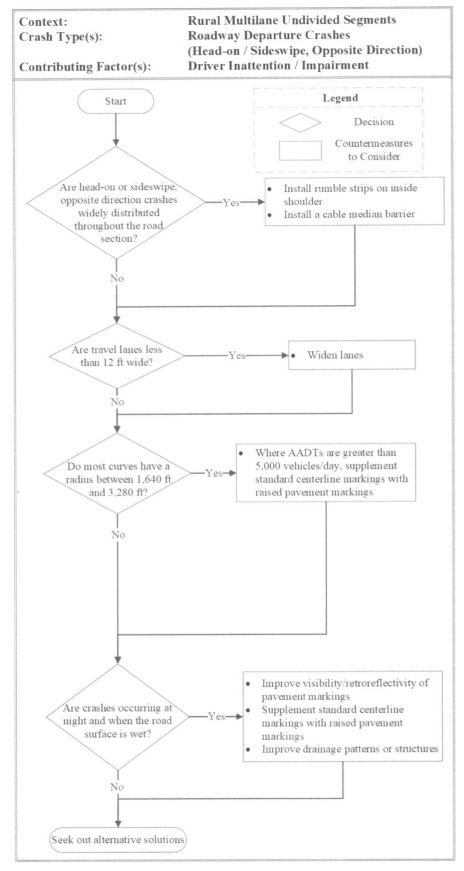

Figure 39.   Rural multilane undivided segments; roadway departure crashes (head-on/sideswipe, opposite direction); driver inattention/ impairment (Source for information on supplementing standard centerline markings: Brewer and Bedsole, 2015; Albin et al., 2016).

Context: **Rural Multilane Undivided Segments**
Crash Type(s):   **Roadway Departure Crashes**
                            (Head-on / Sideswipe, Opposite Direction)
Contributing Factor(s):   **Roadside Design**

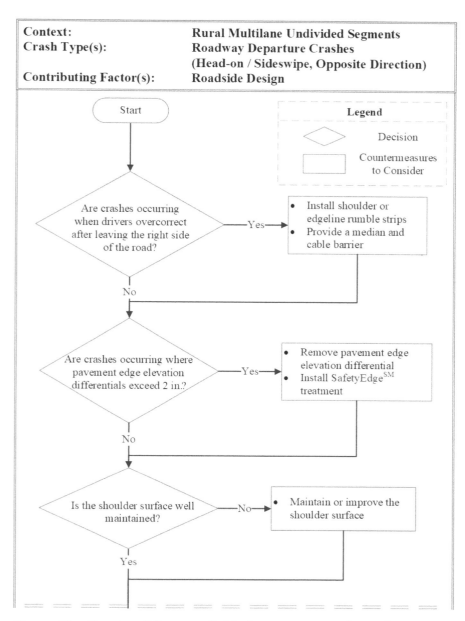

Figure 40.   Rural multilane undivided segments; roadway departure crashes (head-on/sideswipe, opposite direction); roadside design.

(continued on next page)

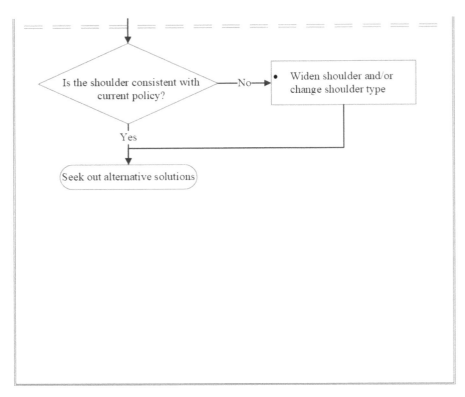

Figure 40.   (Continued).

Context: **Rural Multilane Undivided Segments**
Crash Type(s):   **Roadway Departure Crashes (Head-on /**
                            Sideswipe, Opposite Direction)
Contributing Factor(s):   **Speed / Curvature / Guidance**

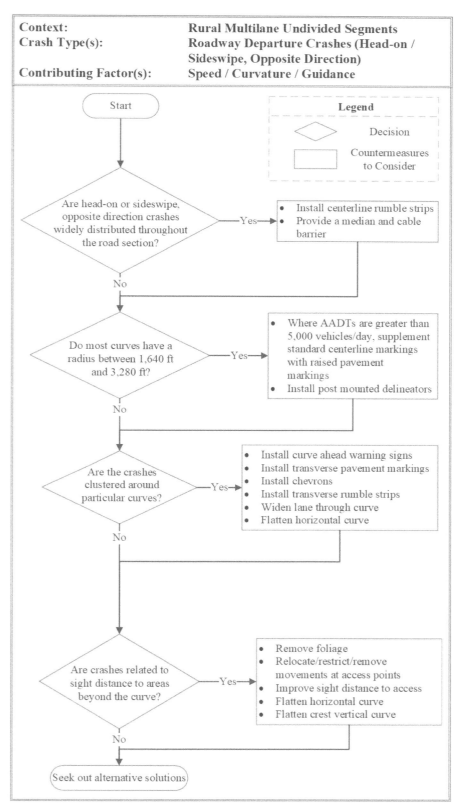

Figure 41.   Rural multilane undivided segments; roadway departure crashes (head-on/sideswipe, opposite direction); speed/curvature/ guidance (Source for information on supplementing standard centerline markings: Brewer and Bedsole, 2015; Albin et al., 2016).

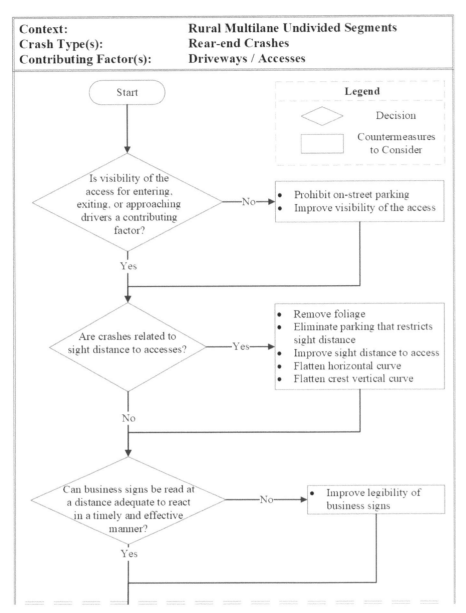

Figure 42.   Rural multilane undivided segments; rear-end crashes; driveways/accesses.

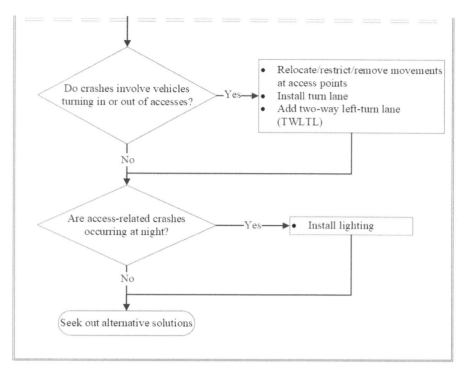

Figure 42.   (Continued).

Context: **Rural Multilane Undivided Segments**
Crash Type(s):   **Pedestrian Crashes**
Contributing Factor(s):   **Dart-dash / Midblock / Along the Road**

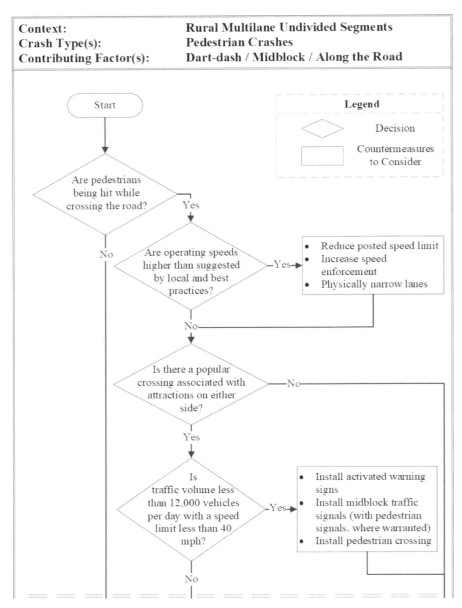

Figure 43.   Rural multilane undivided segments; pedestrian crashes; dart-dash/midblock/along the road.

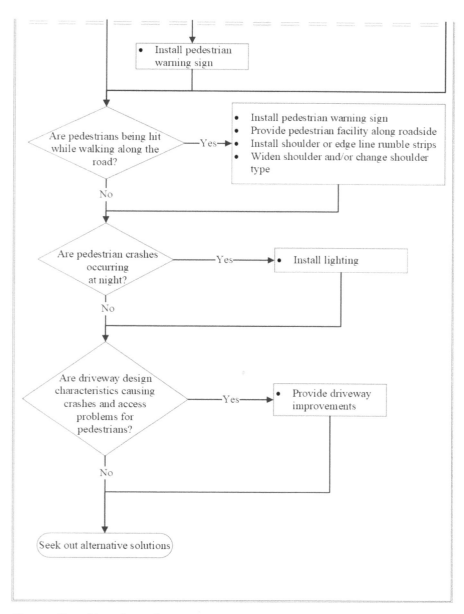

Figure 43.   (Continued).

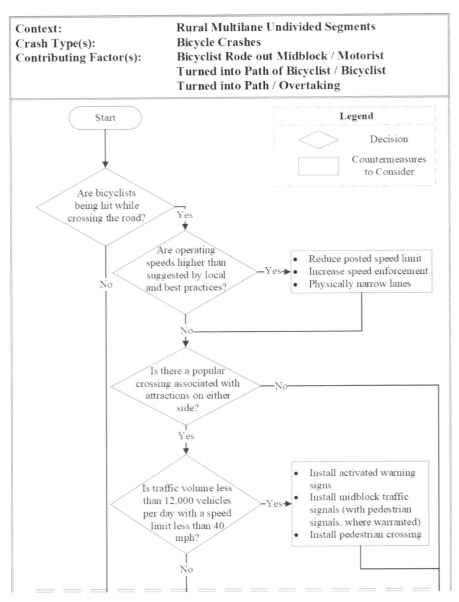

Figure 44. Rural multilane undivided segments; bicycle crashes; bicyclist rode out midblock/motorist turned into path of bicyclist/bicyclist turned into path/overtaking.

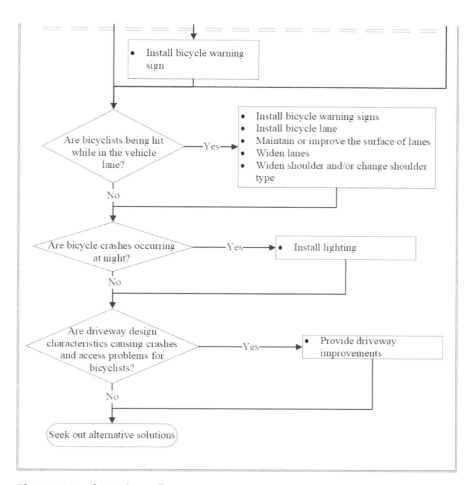

Figure 44. (Continued).

10.5 Rural Multilane Divided Segments

Figures 45 to 55 present the decision trees for rural multilane divided segments.

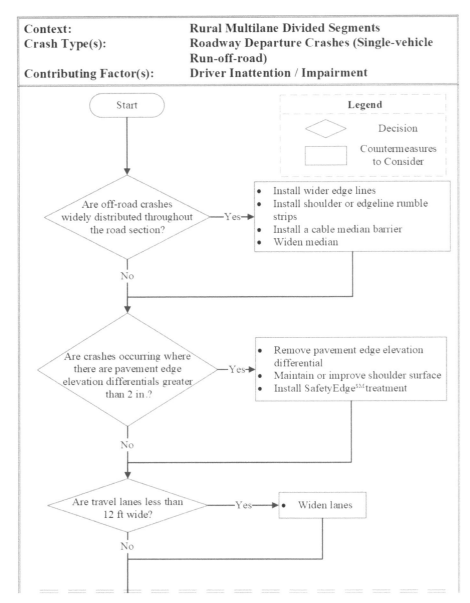

Figure 45.   Rural multilane divided segments; roadway departure crashes (single-vehicle run-off-road); driver inattention/impairment.

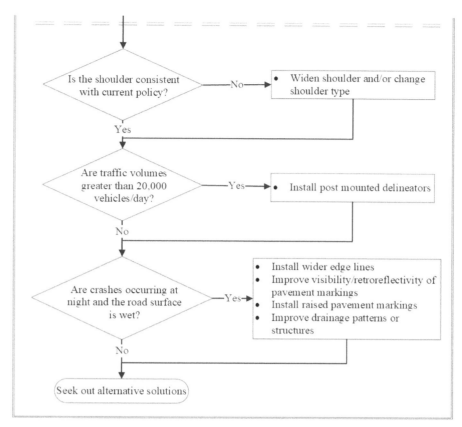

Figure 45.   (Continued).

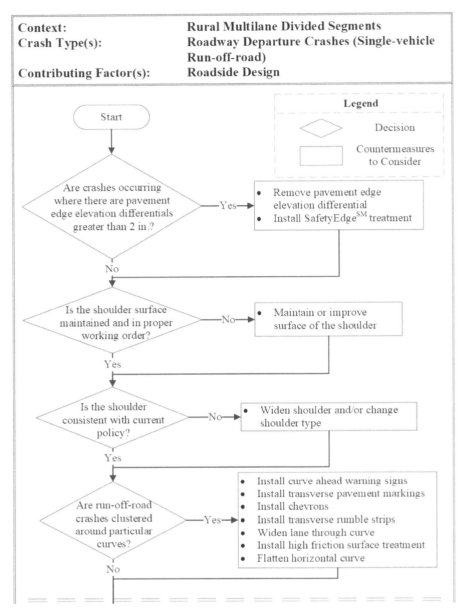

Figure 46. Rural multilane divided segments; roadway departure crashes (single-vehicle run-off-road); roadside design.

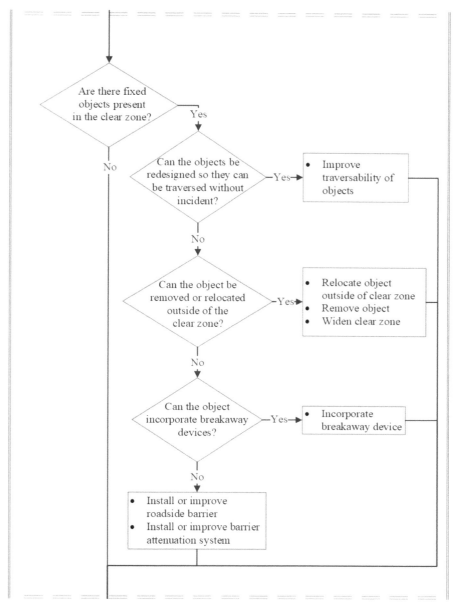

Figure 46.   (Continued).

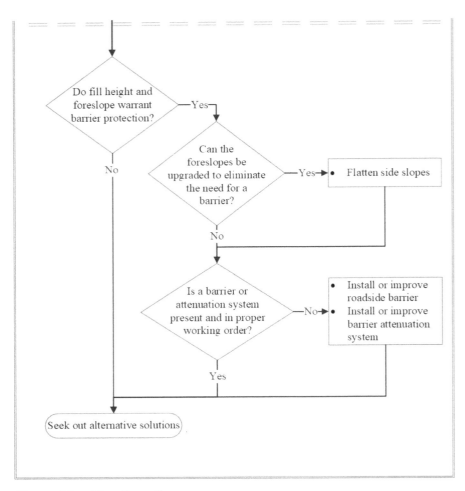

Figure 46.   (Continued).

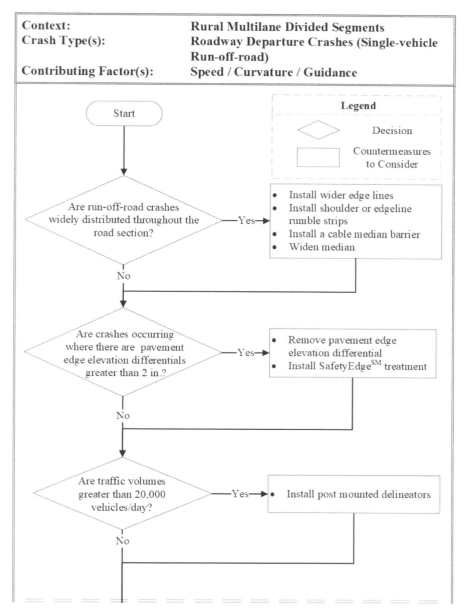

Figure 47.   Rural multilane divided segments; roadway departure crashes (single-vehicle run-off-road); speed/curvature/guidance.

(continued on next page)

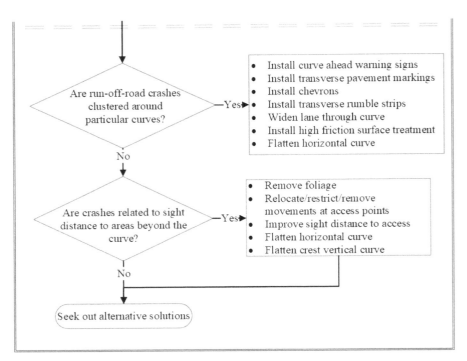

Figure 47. *(Continued).*

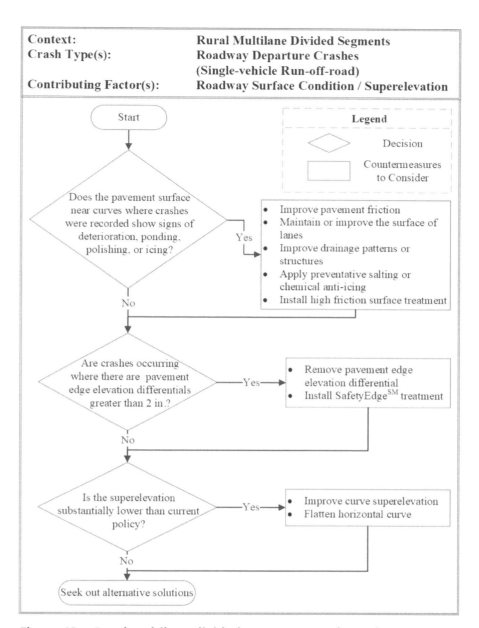

Figure 48.   Rural multilane divided segments; roadway departure crashes (single-vehicle run-off-road); roadway surface condition/ superelevation.

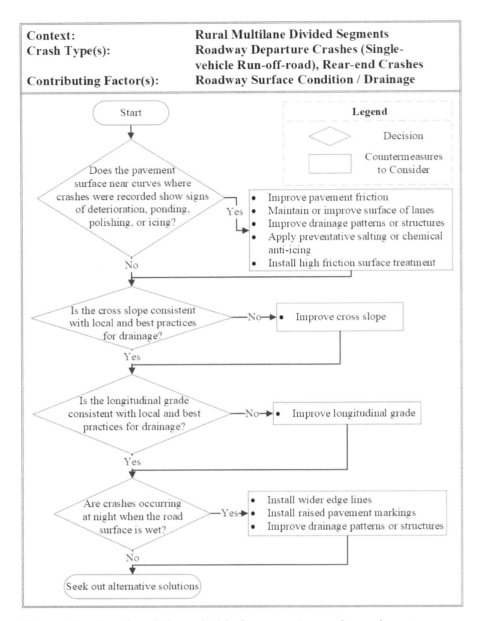

Figure 49.   Rural multilane divided segments; roadway departure crashes (single-vehicle run-off-road), rear-end crashes; roadway surface condition/drainage.

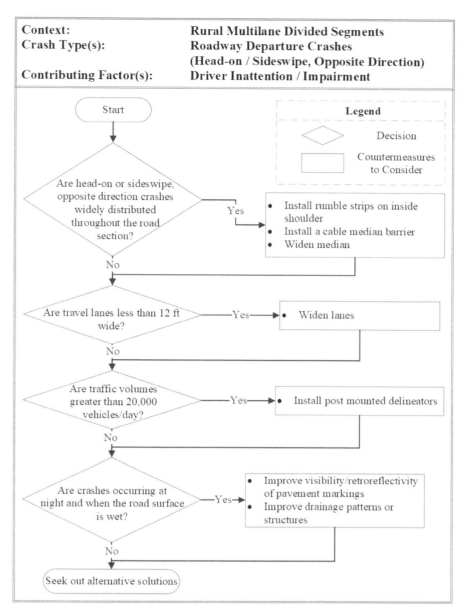

Figure 50.   Rural multilane divided segments; roadway departure crashes (head-on/sideswipe, opposite direction); driver inattention/ impairment.

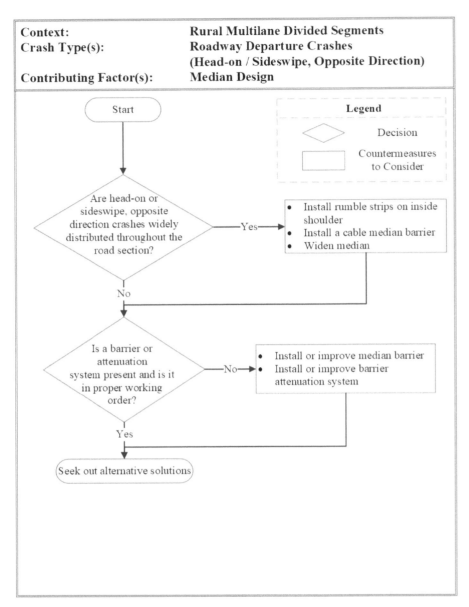

Figure 51.   Rural multilane divided segments; roadway departure crashes (head-on/sideswipe, opposite direction); median design.

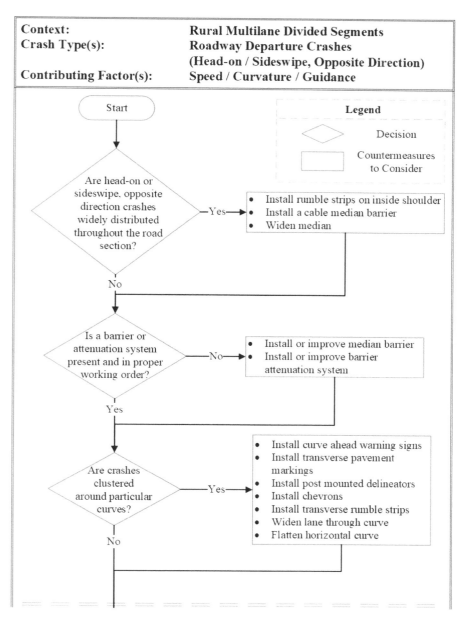

Figure 52.   Rural multilane divided segments; roadway departure crashes (head-on/sideswipe, opposite direction); speed/curvature/guidance.

(continued on next page)

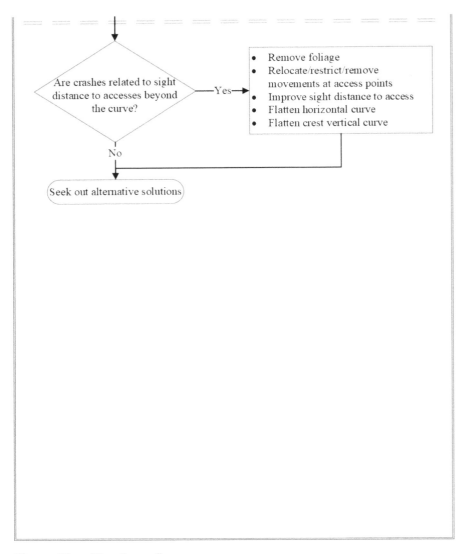

Figure 52. *(Continued).*

Context: **Rural Multilane Divided Segments**
Crash Type(s):   **Rear-end Crashes**
Contributing Factor(s): **Driveways / Accesses**

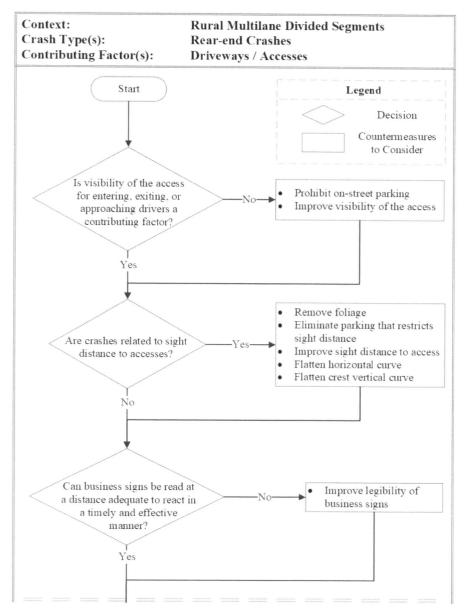

Figure 53.   Rural multilane divided segments; rear-end crashes; driveways/accesses.

(continued on next page)

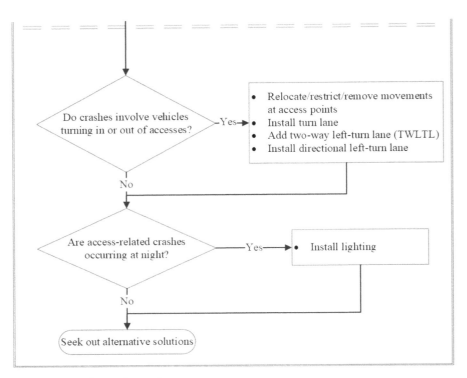

Figure 53.   (Continued).

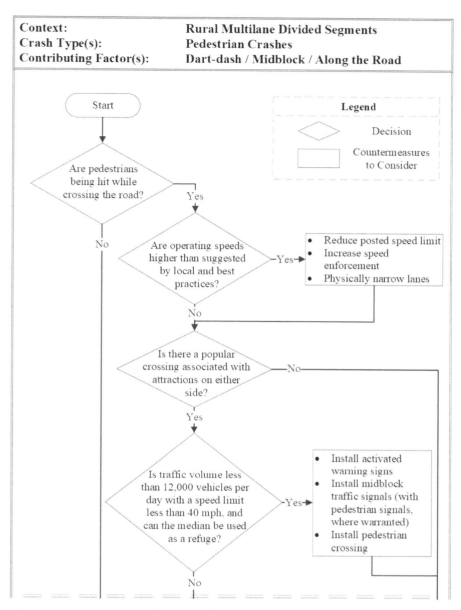

Context: **Rural Multilane Divided Segments**
Crash Type(s):   **Pedestrian Crashes**
Contributing Factor(s):   **Dart-dash / Midblock / Along the Road**

Figure 54. Rural multilane divided segments; pedestrian crashes; dart-dash/midblock/along the road.

(continued on next page)

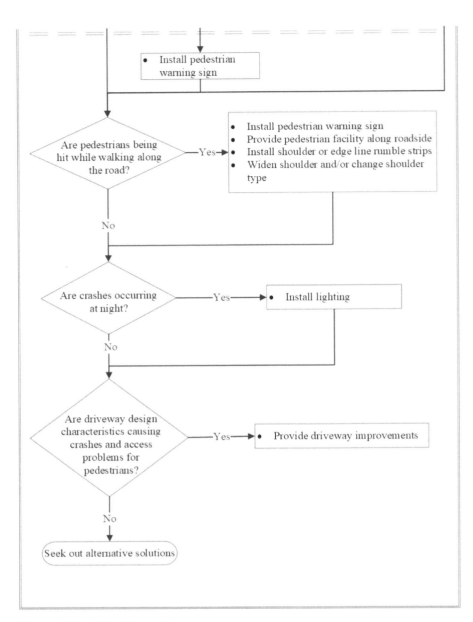

Figure 54.   (Continued).

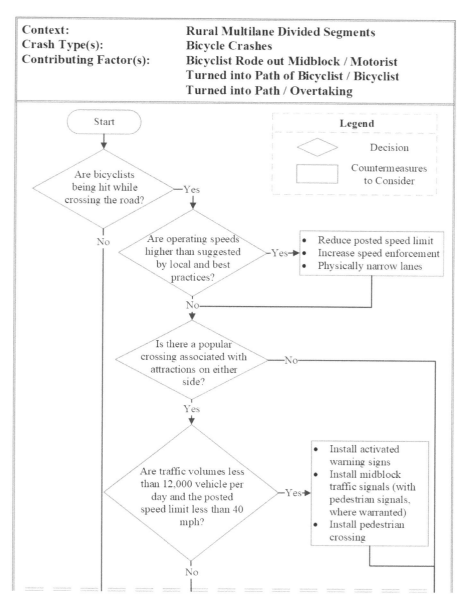

Context: Rural Multilane Divided Segments
Crash Type(s): Bicycle Crashes
Contributing Factor(s): Bicyclist Rode out Midblock / Motorist Turned into Path of Bicyclist / Bicyclist Turned into Path / Overtaking

Figure 55.   Rural multilane divided segments; bicycle crashes; bicyclist rode out midblock/motorist turned into path of bicyclist/bicyclist turned into path/overtaking.

(continued on next page)

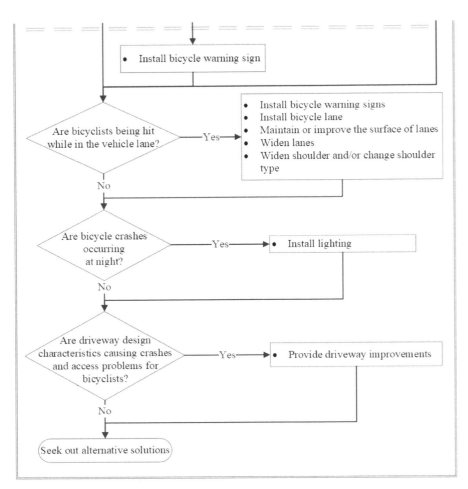

Figure 55.   (Continued).

10.6 Urban Two-lane Segments

Figures 56 to 63 present the decision trees for urban two-lane segments.

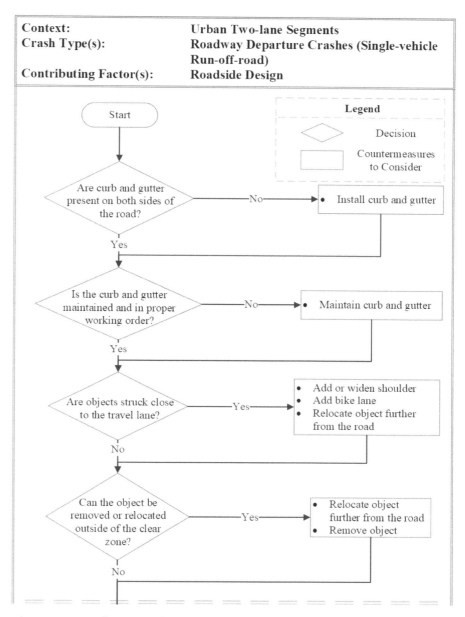

Figure 56. Urban two-lane segments; roadway departure crashes (single-vehicle run-off-road); roadside design.

(continued on next page)

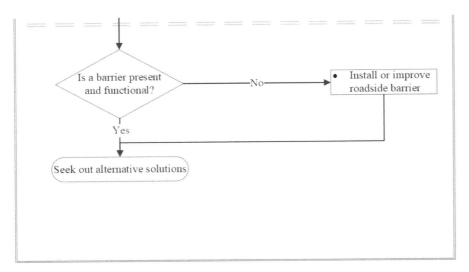

Figure 56. *(Continued).*

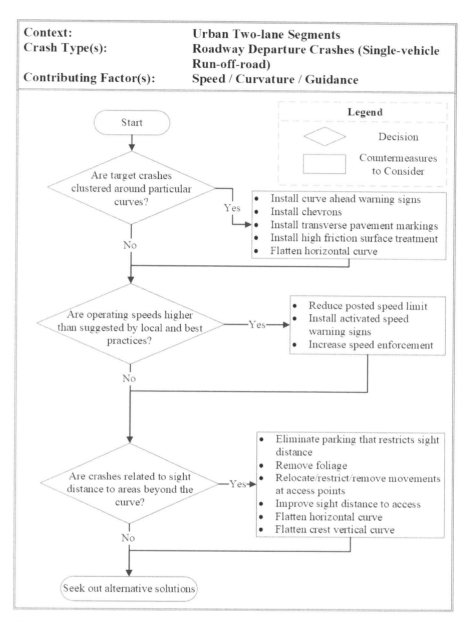

Figure 57.   Urban two-lane segments; roadway departure crashes (single-vehicle run-off-road); speed/curvature/guidance.

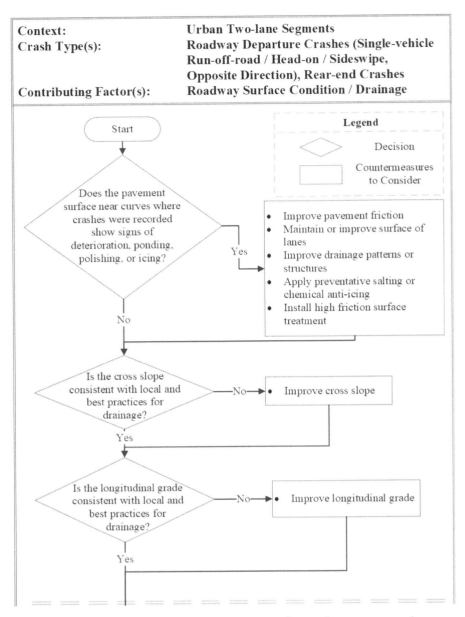

Figure 58. Urban two-lane segments; roadway departure crashes (single-vehicle run-off-road/head-on/rear-end/sideswipe, opposite direction), rear-end crashes; roadway surface condition/drainage.

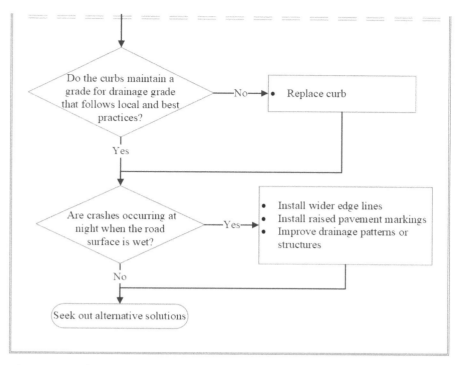

Figure 58.   (Continued).

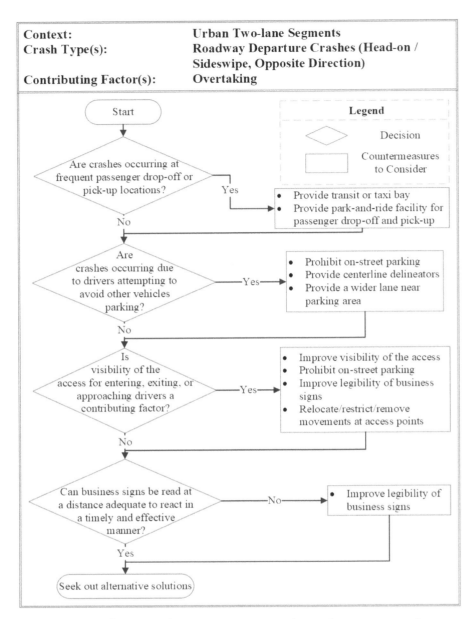

Figure 59. Urban two-lane segments; roadway departure crashes (head-on/sideswipe, opposite direction); overtaking.

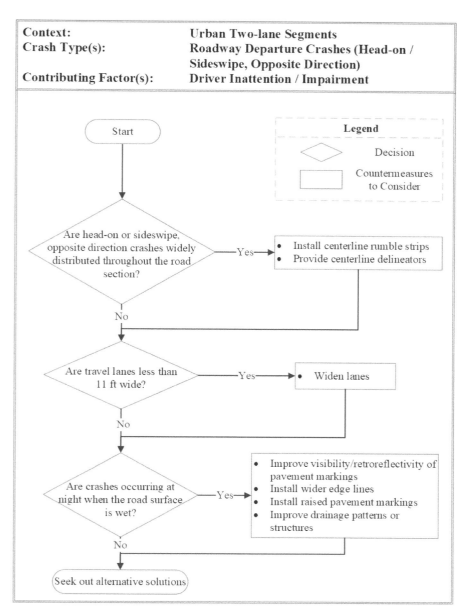

Figure 60.   Urban two-lane segments; roadway departure crashes (head-on/sideswipe, opposite direction); driver inattention/impairment.

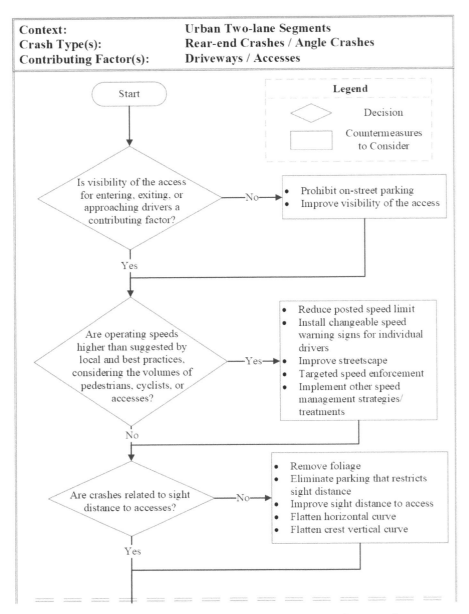

Figure 61.   Urban two-lane segments; rear-end crashes/angle crashes; driveways/accesses.

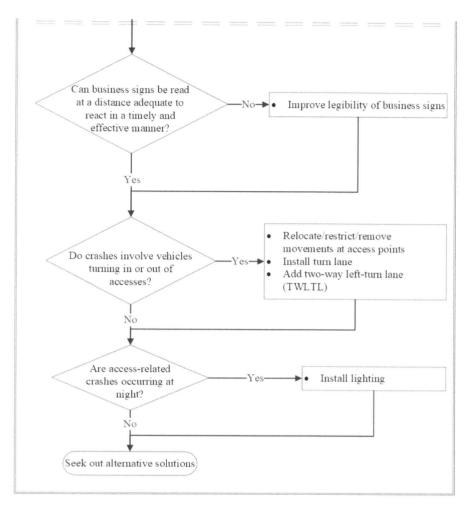

Figure 61. *(Continued).*

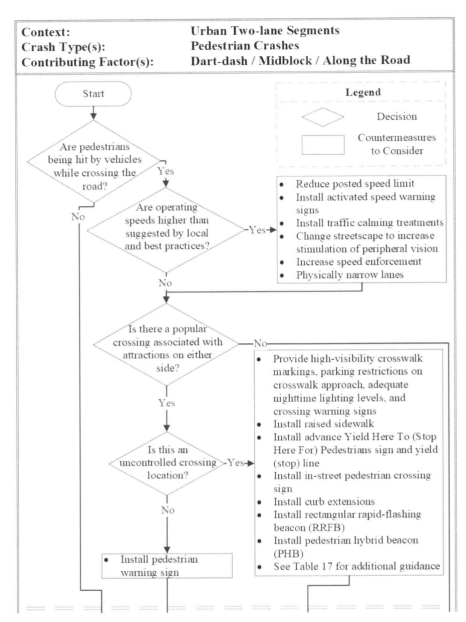

Figure 62. *Urban two-lane segments; pedestrian crashes; dart-dash/ midblock/along the road.*

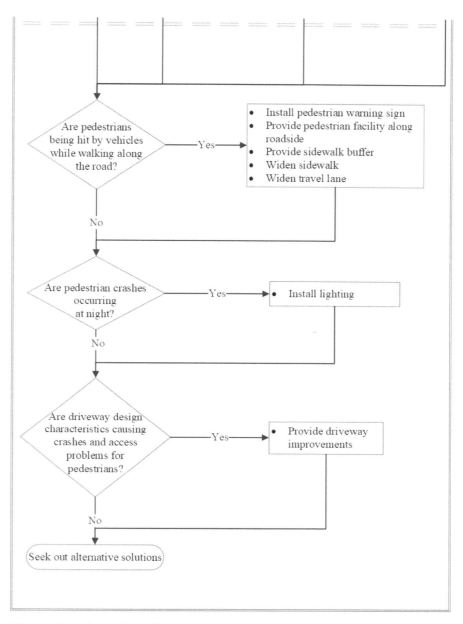

Figure 62.   (Continued).

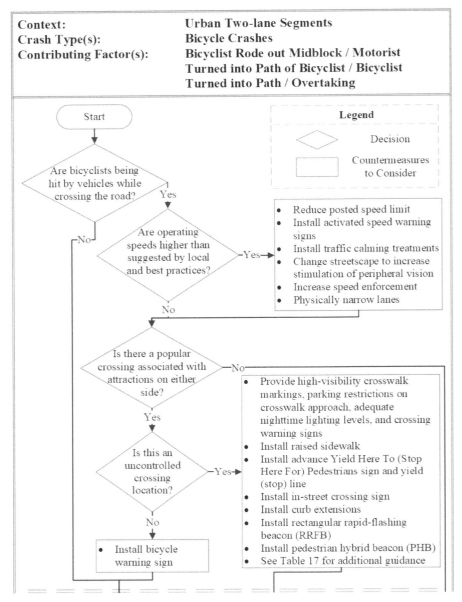

Figure 63. Urban two-lane segments; bicycle crashes; bicyclist rode out midblock/motorist turned into path of bicyclist/bicyclist turned into path/overtaking.

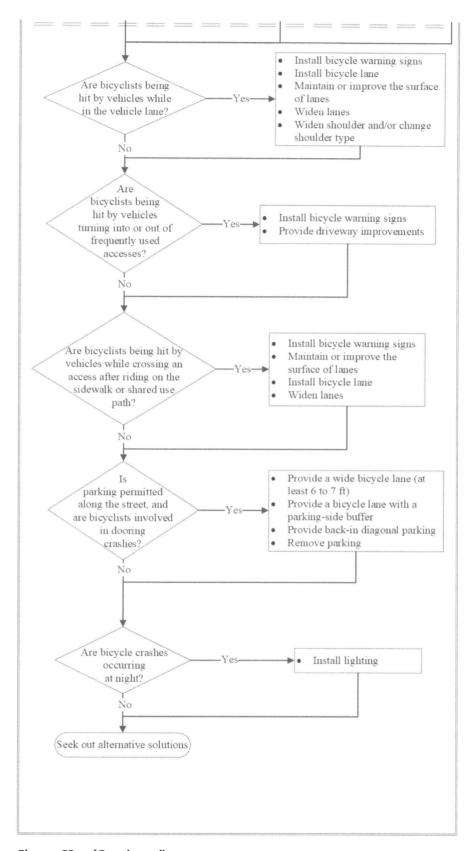

Are bicyclists being hit by vehicles while in the vehicle lane?

—Yes→
- Install bicycle warning signs
- Install bicycle lane
- Maintain or improve the surface of lanes
- Widen lanes
- Widen shoulder and/or change shoulder type

No

Are bicyclists being hit by vehicles turning into or out of frequently used accesses?

—Yes→
- Install bicycle warning signs
- Provide driveway improvements

No

Are bicyclists being hit by vehicles while crossing an access after riding on the sidewalk or shared use path?

—Yes→
- Install bicycle warning signs
- Maintain or improve the surface of lanes
- Install bicycle lane
- Widen lanes

No

Is parking permitted along the street, and are bicyclists involved in dooring crashes?

—Yes→
- Provide a wide bicycle lane (at least 6 to 7 ft)
- Provide a bicycle lane with a parking-side buffer
- Provide back-in diagonal parking
- Remove parking

No

Are bicycle crashes occurring at night?

—Yes→
- Install lighting

No

Seek out alternative solutions

Figure 63.   (Continued).

10.7 Urban Multilane Undivided Segments

Figures 64 to 72 present the decision trees for urban multilane undivided segments.

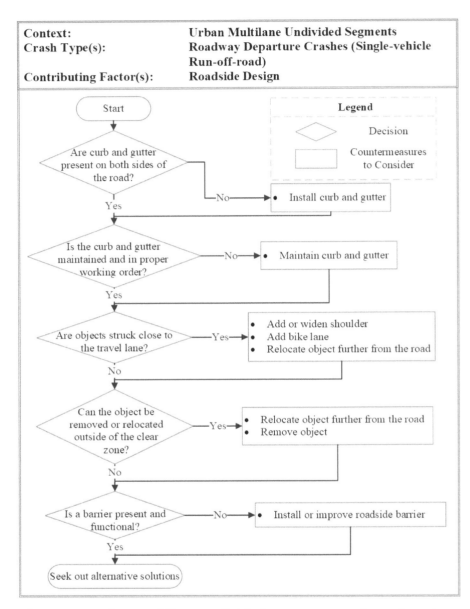

Figure 64. *Urban multilane undivided segments; roadway departure crashes (single-vehicle run-off-road); roadside design.*

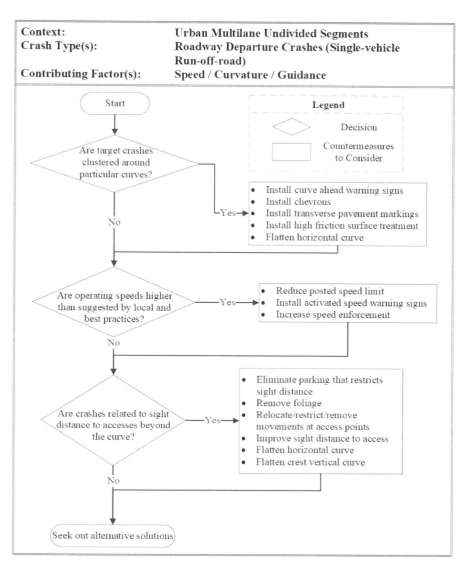

Figure 65.   Urban multilane undivided segments; roadway departure crashes (single-vehicle run-off-road); speed/curvature/guidance.

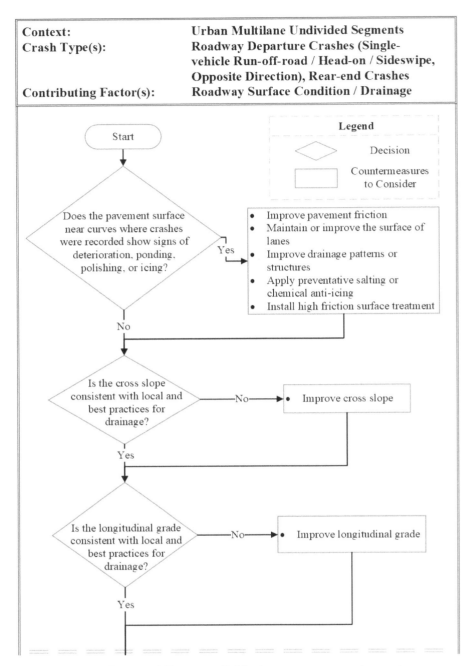

Figure 66. Urban multilane undivided segments; roadway departure crashes (single-vehicle run-off-road/head-on/sideswipe, opposite direction), rear-end crashes; roadway surface condition/drainage.

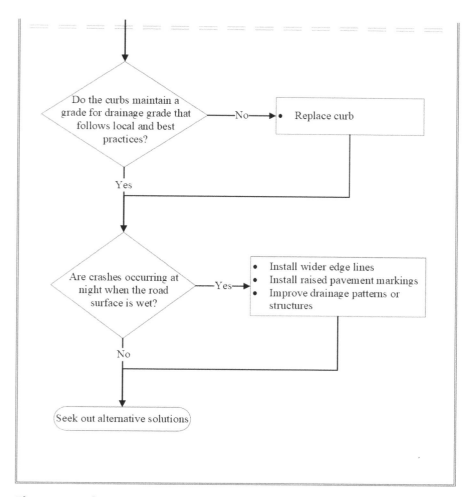

Figure 66.   (Continued).

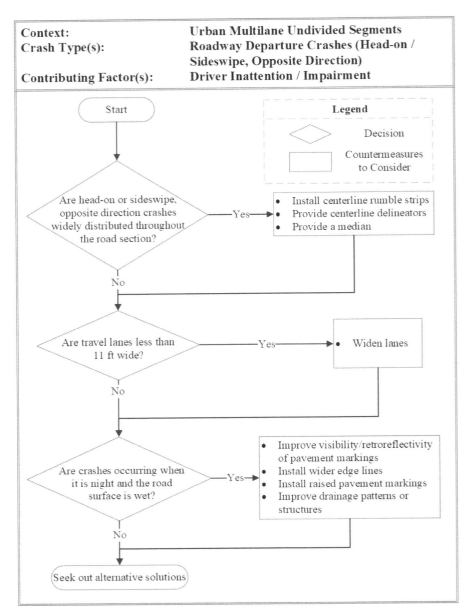

Context:	Urban Multilane Undivided Segments
Crash Type(s):	Roadway Departure Crashes (Head-on / Sideswipe, Opposite Direction)
Contributing Factor(s):	Driver Inattention / Impairment

Figure 67. Urban multilane undivided segments; roadway departure crashes (head-on/sideswipe, opposite direction); driver inattention/impairment.

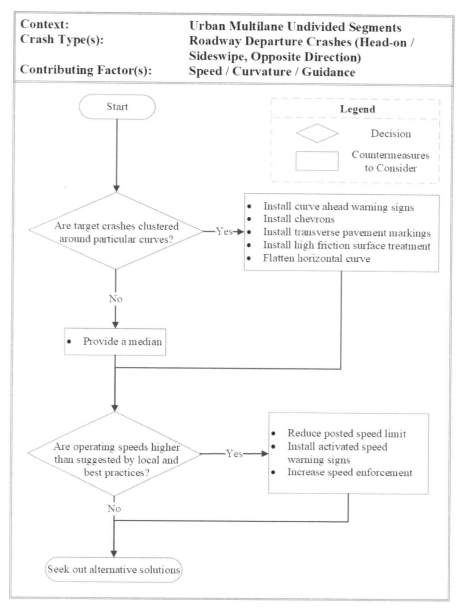

Figure 68. Urban multilane undivided segments; roadway departure crashes (head-on/sideswipe, opposite direction); speed/curvature/ guidance.

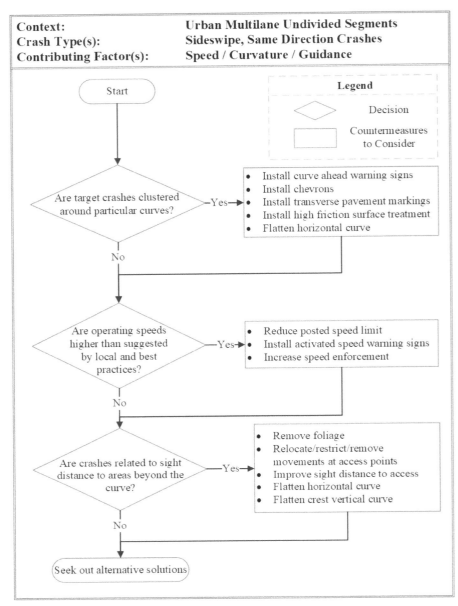

Figure 69. *Urban multilane undivided segments; sideswipe, same direction crashes; speed/curvature/guidance.*

Context: **Urban Multilane Undivided Segments**
Crash Type(s):   **Rear-end Crashes / Angle Crashes /**
                                  Sideswipe, Same Direction Crashes
Contributing Factor(s):   **Driveways / Accesses**

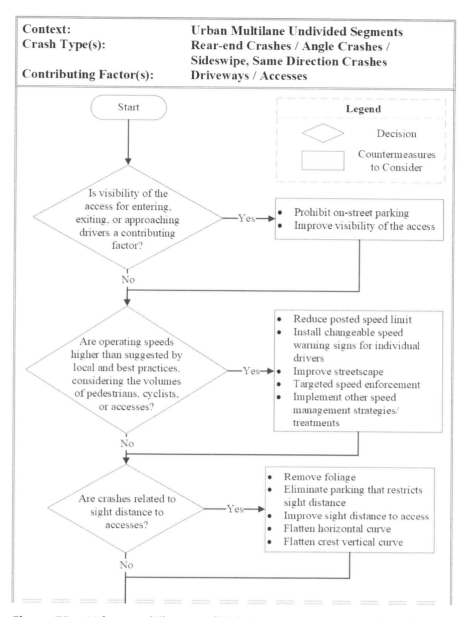

Figure 70.   Urban multilane undivided segments; rear-end crashes/ angle crashes/sideswipe, same direction crashes, driveway/accesses.

(continued on next page)

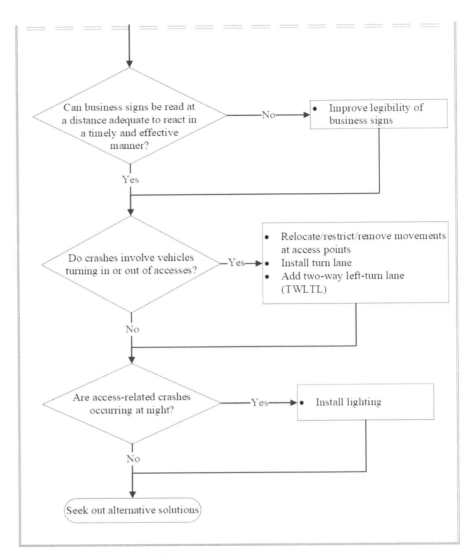

Figure 70. *(Continued).*

Context:	Urban Multilane Undivided Segments
Crash Type(s):	Pedestrian Crashes
Contributing Factor(s):	Dart-dash / Midblock / Along the Road

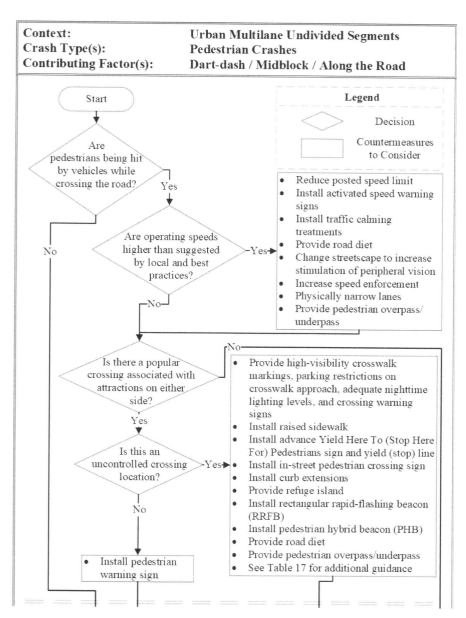

Figure 71.   *Urban multilane undivided segments; pedestrian crashes; dart-dash/midblock/along the road.*

(continued on next page)

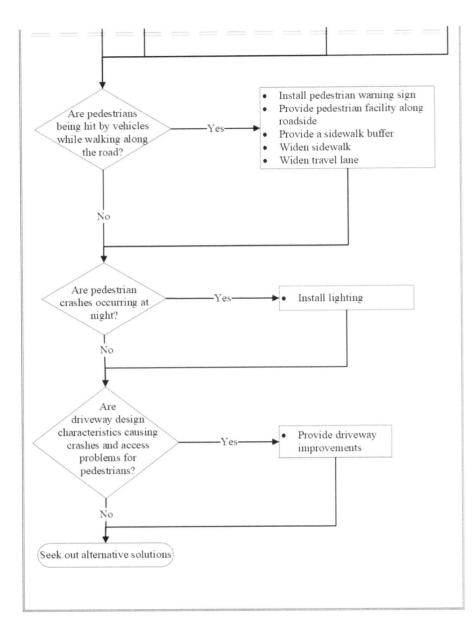

Figure 71.   (Continued).

Context: **Urban Multilane Undivided Segments**
Crash Type(s):   **Bicycle Crashes**
Contributing Factor(s):   **Bicyclist Rode out Midblock / Motorist Turned into Path / Bicyclist Turned into Path / Overtaking**

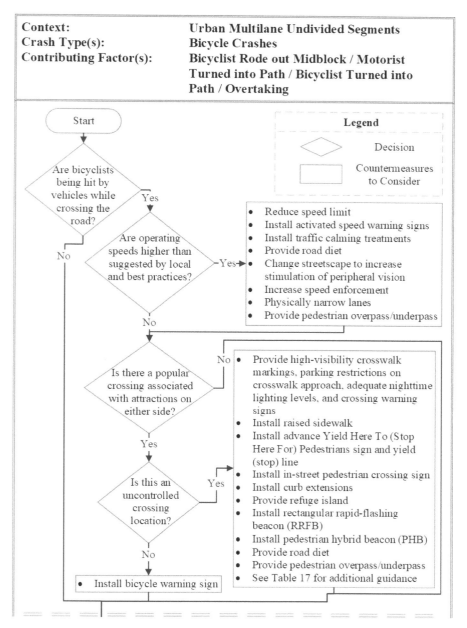

Figure 72.   Urban multilane undivided segments; bicycle crashes; bicyclist rode out midblock/motorist turned into path/bicyclist turned into path/overtaking.

(continued on next page)

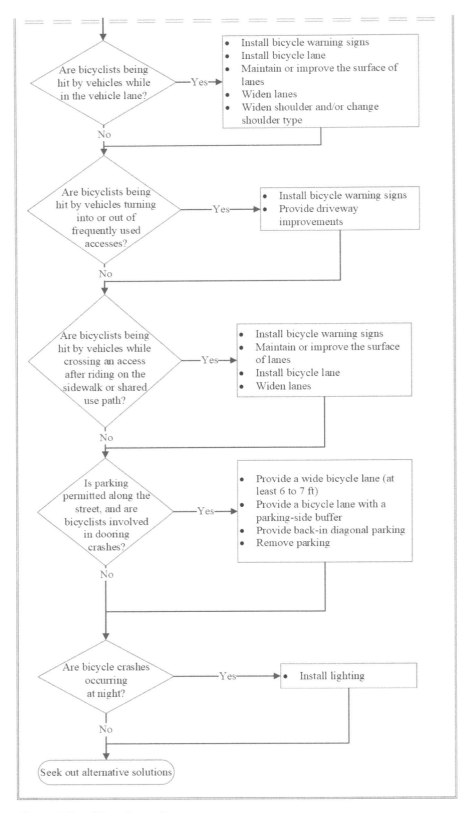

Figure 72. (Continued).

10.8 Urban Multilane Divided Segments

Figures 73 to 77 present the decision trees for urban multilane divided segments.

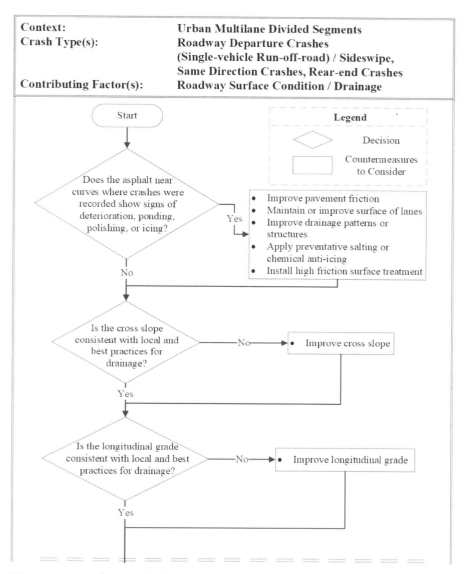

Figure 73.   Urban multilane divided segments; roadway departure crashes (single-vehicle run-off-road)/sideswipe, same direction crashes, rear-end crashes; roadway surface condition/drainage.

(continued on next page)

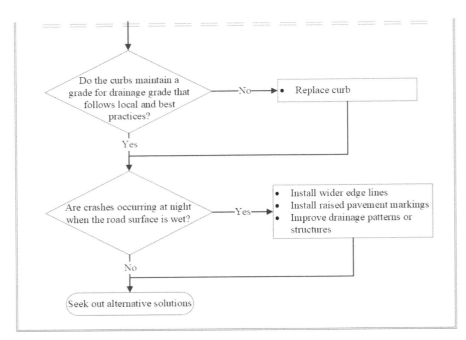

Figure 73. *(Continued).*

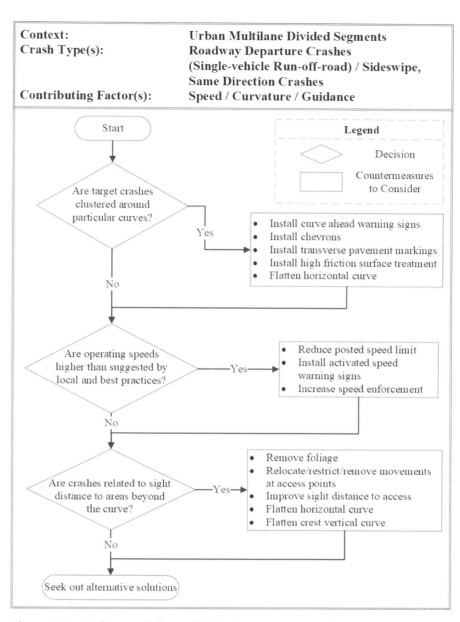

Figure 74.   Urban multilane divided segments; roadway departure crashes (single-vehicle run-off-road)/sideswipe, same direction crashes; speed/curvature/guidance.

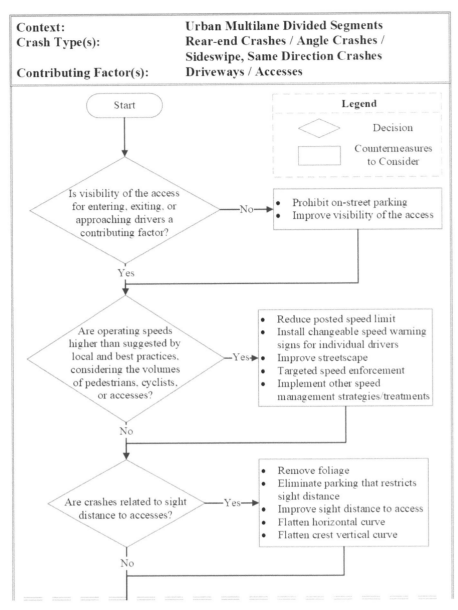

Figure 75. Urban multilane divided segments; rear-end crashes/angle crashes/sideswipe, same direction crashes; driveways/accesses.

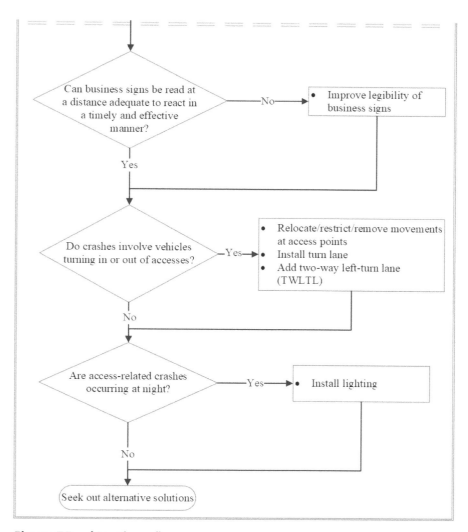

Figure 75.   (Continued).

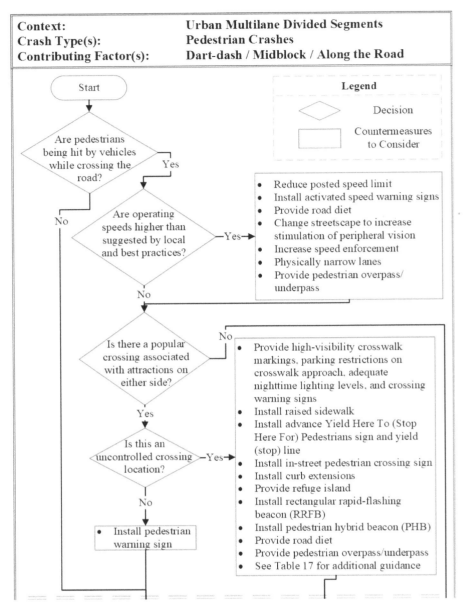

Figure 76.   Urban multilane divided segments; pedestrian crashes; dart-dash/midblock/along the road.

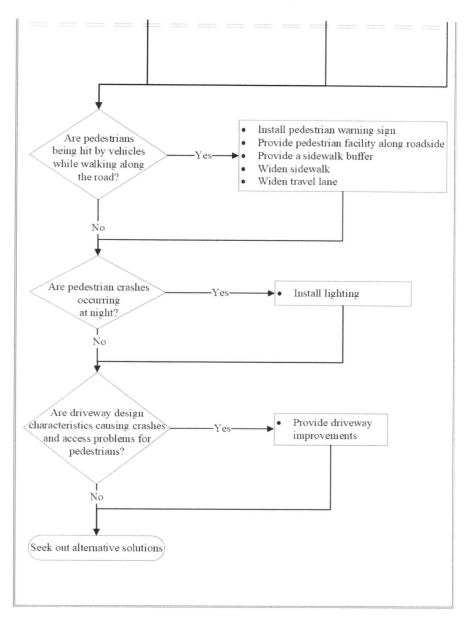

Figure 76.   (Continued).

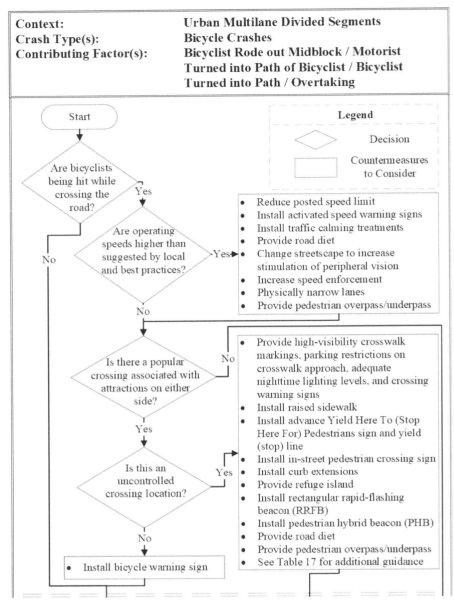

Figure 77. Urban multilane divided segments; bicycle crashes; bicyclist rode out midblock/motorist turned into path of bicyclist/bicyclist turned into path/overtaking.

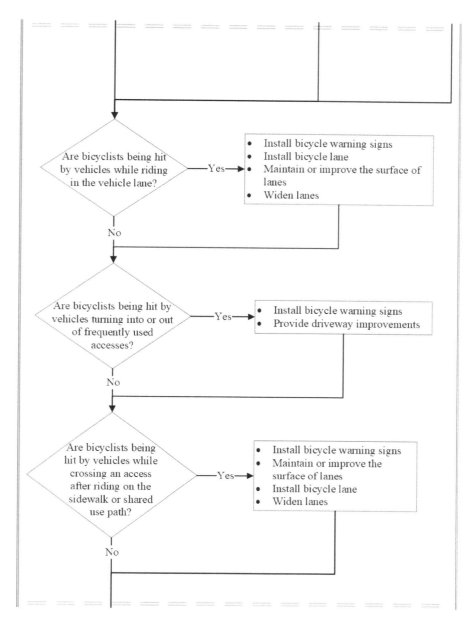

Figure 77. (Continued).

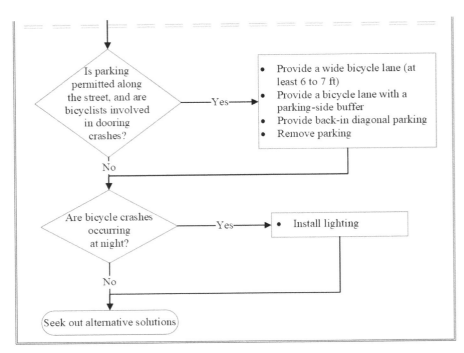

Figure 77. *(Continued).*

10.9 Rural and Urban Signalized Intersections

Figures 78 to 93 present the decision trees for rural and urban signalized intersections.

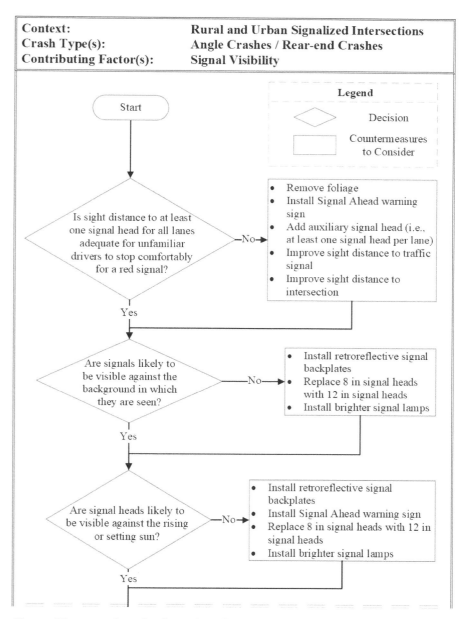

Figure 78.   Rural and urban signalized intersections; angle crashes, rear-end crashes; signal visibility.

(continued on next page)

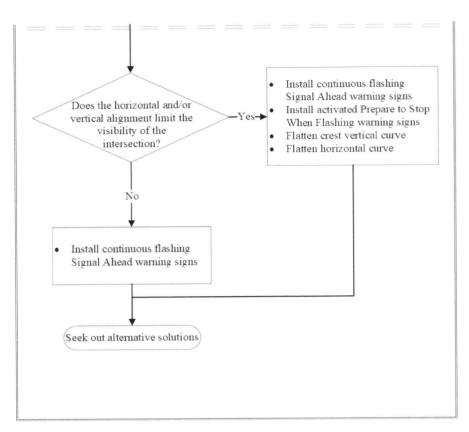

Figure 78. (Continued).

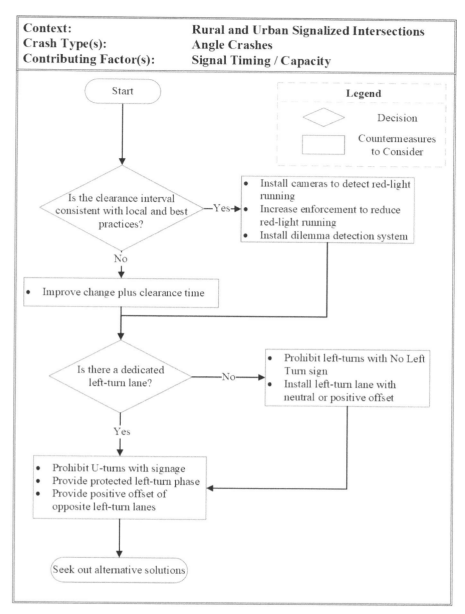

Figure 79.   Rural and urban signalized intersections; angle crashes; signal timing/capacity.

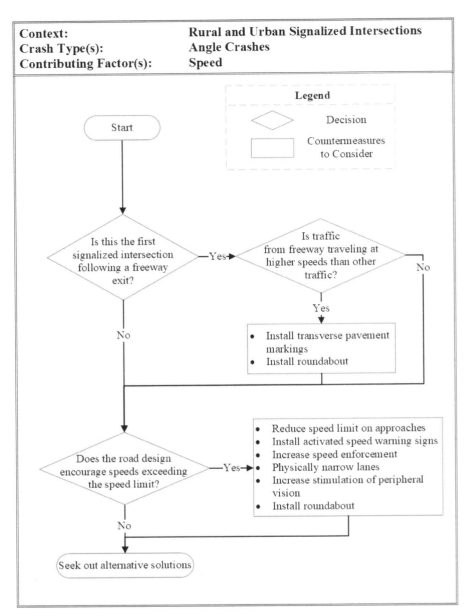

Figure 80. Rural and urban signalized intersections; angle crashes; speed.

Context: **Rural and Urban Signalized Intersections**
Crash Type(s): **Angle Crashes / Rear-end Crashes**
Contributing Factor(s): **Pavement Friction**

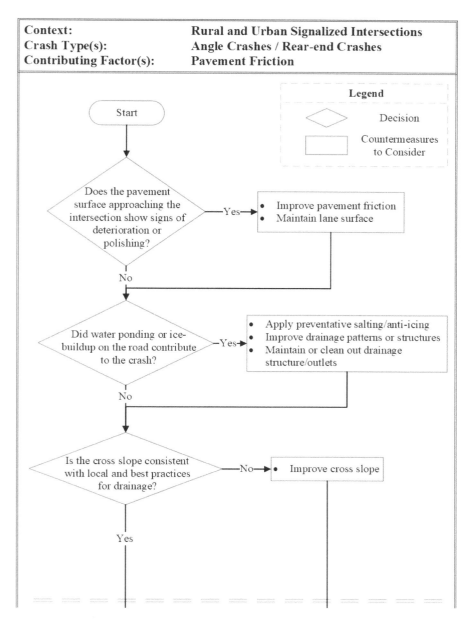

Figure 81. Rural and urban signalized intersections; angle crashes, rear-end crashes; pavement friction.

(continued on next page)

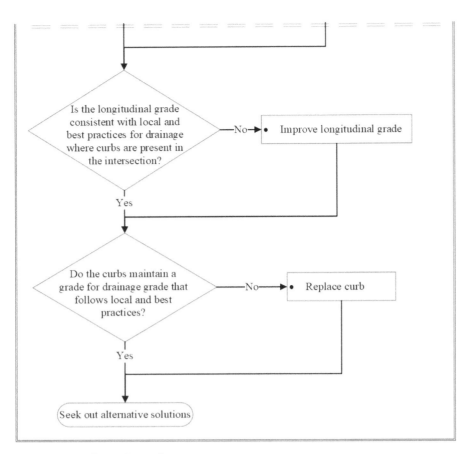

Figure 81.   (Continued).

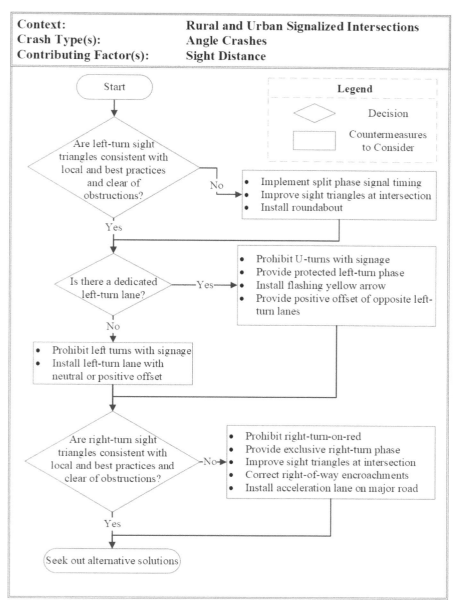

Context: **Rural and Urban Signalized Intersections**
Crash Type(s):   **Angle Crashes**
Contributing Factor(s):   **Sight Distance**

Figure 82.   Rural and urban signalized intersections; angle crashes; sight distance.

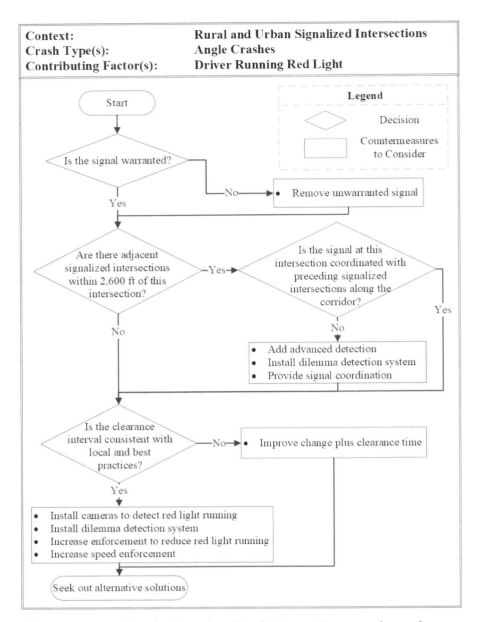

Figure 83. Rural and urban signalized intersections; angle crashes; driver running red light.

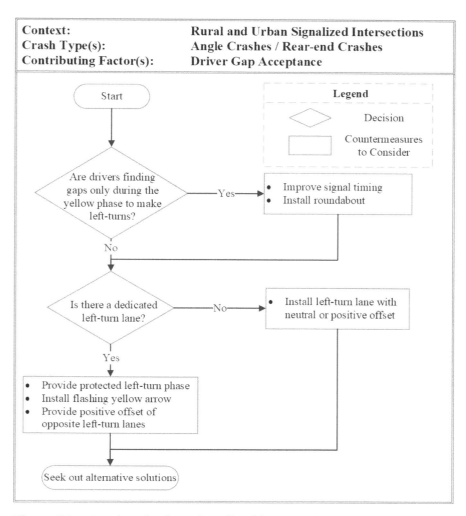

Figure 84.   Rural and urban signalized intersections; angle crashes, rear-end crashes; driver gap acceptance.

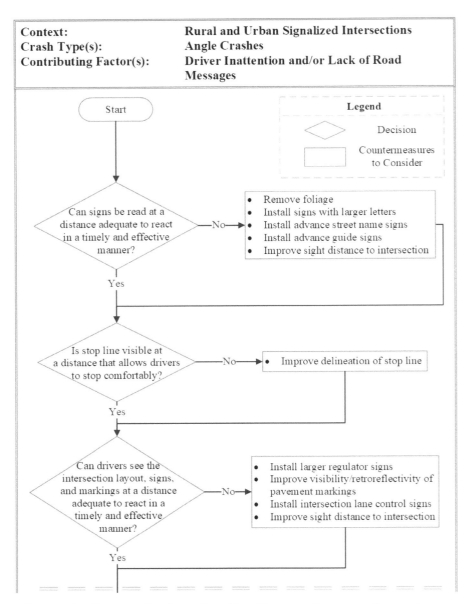

Context: Rural and Urban Signalized Intersections
Crash Type(s): Angle Crashes
Contributing Factor(s): Driver Inattention and/or Lack of Road Messages

Figure 85. Rural and urban signalized intersections; angle crashes; driver inattention and/or lack of road messages.

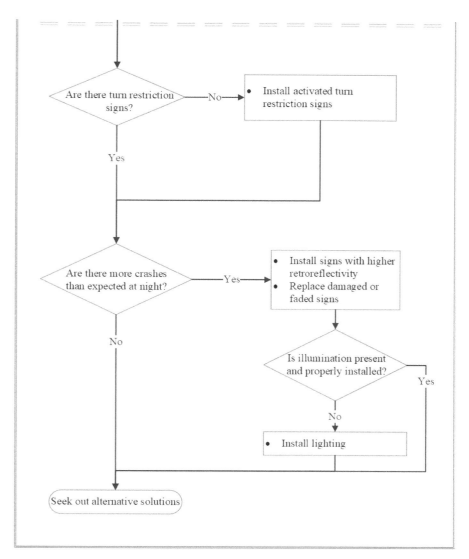

Figure 85.   (Continued).

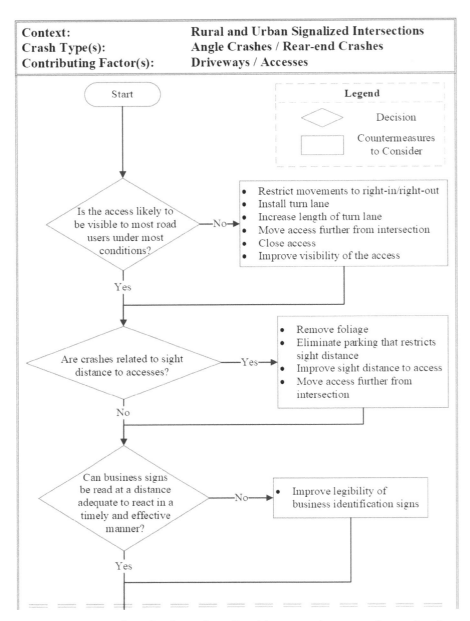

Figure 86. Rural and urban signalized intersections; angle crashes/ rear-end crashes; driveways/accesses.

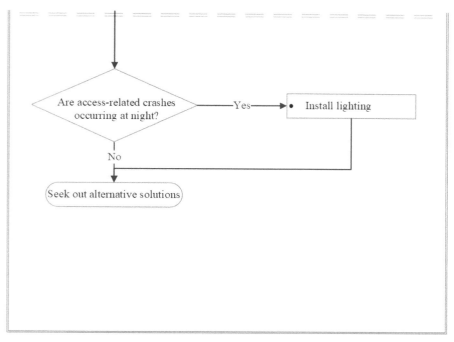

Figure 86. *(Continued).*

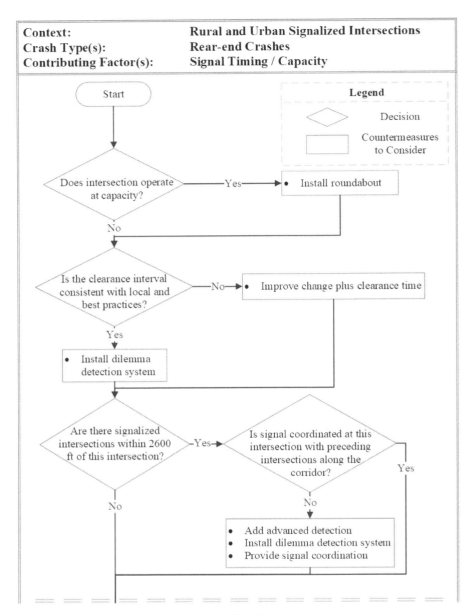

Figure 87. Rural and urban signalized intersections; rear-end crashes; signal timing/capacity.

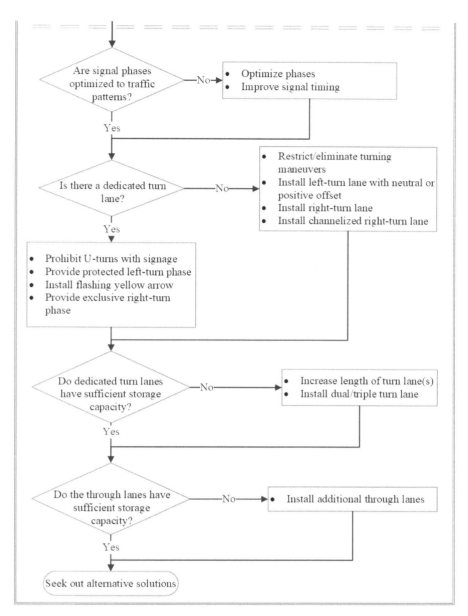

Figure 87.   (Continued).

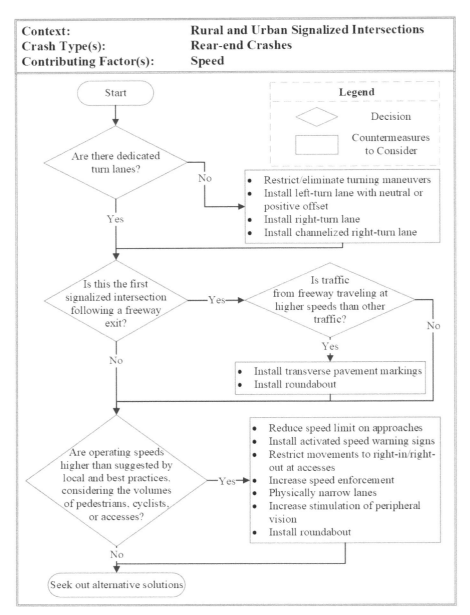

Figure 88. Rural and urban signalized intersections; rear-end crashes; speed.

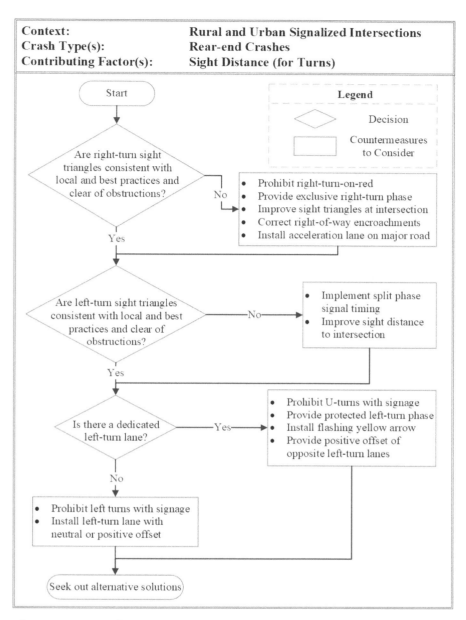

Context: **Rural and Urban Signalized Intersections**
Crash Type(s):   **Rear-end Crashes**
Contributing Factor(s):   **Sight Distance (for Turns)**

Legend

◇ Decision

▢ Countermeasures to Consider

Start

Are right-turn sight triangles consistent with local and best practices and clear of obstructions?

No
- Prohibit right-turn-on-red
- Provide exclusive right-turn phase
- Improve sight triangles at intersection
- Correct right-of-way encroachments
- Install acceleration lane on major road

Yes

Are left-turn sight triangles consistent with local and best practices and clear of obstructions?

No
- Implement split phase signal timing
- Improve sight distance to intersection

Yes

Is there a dedicated left-turn lane?

Yes
- Prohibit U-turns with signage
- Provide protected left-turn phase
- Install flashing yellow arrow
- Provide positive offset of opposite left-turn lanes

No
- Prohibit left turns with signage
- Install left-turn lane with neutral or positive offset

Seek out alternative solutions

Figure 89.   Rural and urban signalized intersections; rear-end crashes; sight distance (for turns).

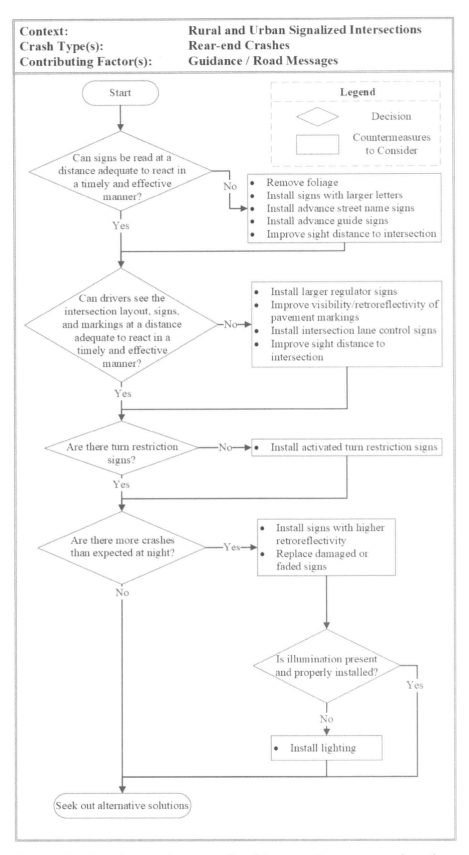

Figure 90.   Rural and urban signalized intersections; rear-end crashes; guidance/road messages.

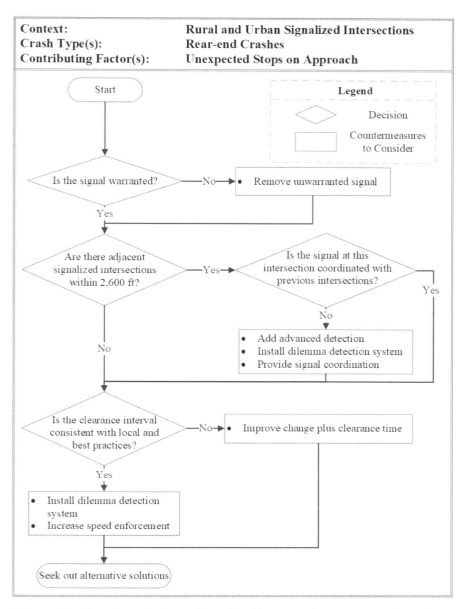

Figure 91.   Rural and urban signalized intersections; rear-end crashes; unexpected stops on approach.

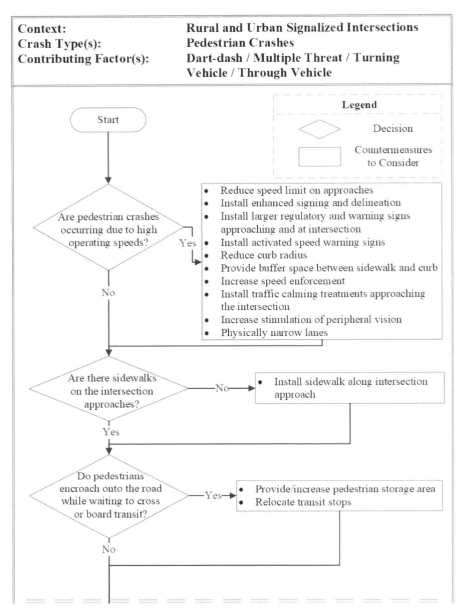

Figure 92. Rural and urban signalized intersections; pedestrian crashes; dart-dash/multiple threat/turning vehicle/through vehicle.

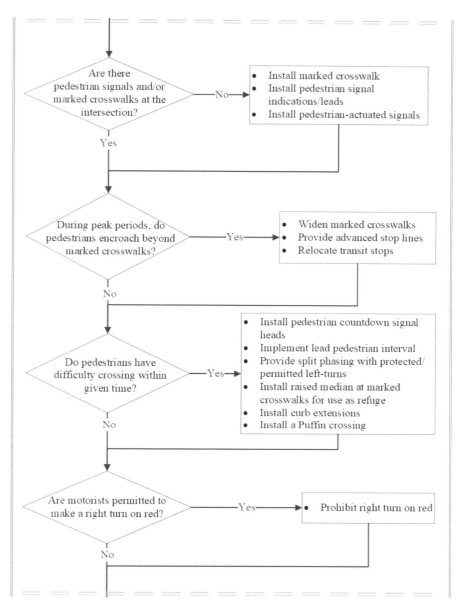

Figure 92. (Continued).

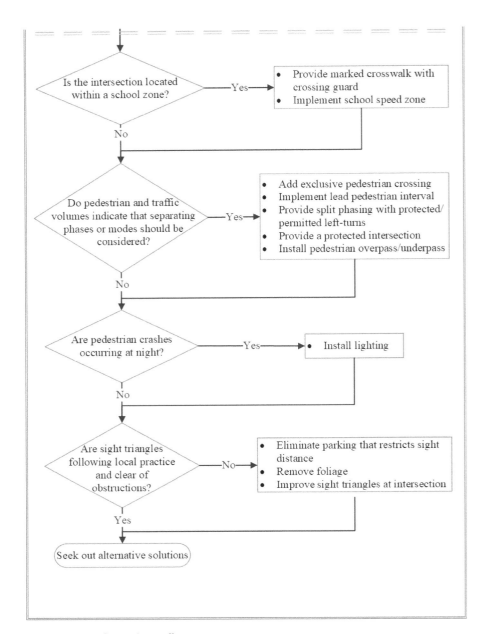

Figure 92. *(Continued).*

Decision Trees to Support Countermeasure Selection **209**

Context: **Rural and Urban Signalized Intersections**
Crash Type(s): **Bicycle Crashes**
Contributing Factor(s): **Motorist Failed to Yield / Bicyclist Failed to Yield / Turning Vehicle**

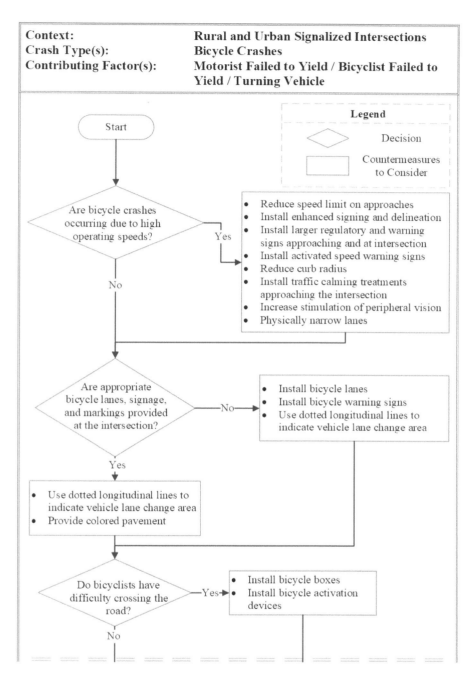

Figure 93. Rural and urban signalized intersections; bicycle crashes; motorist failed to yield/bicyclist failed to yield/turning vehicle.

(continued on next page)

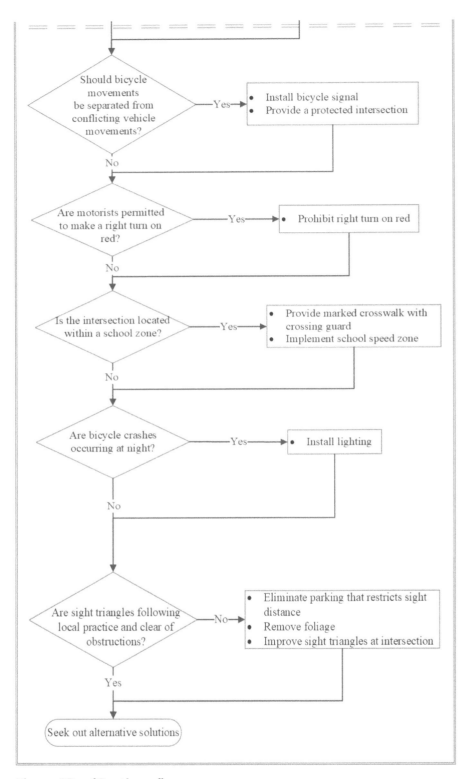

Figure 93.   (Continued).

10.10 Rural and Urban Unsignalized Intersections

Figures 94 to 102 present the decision trees for rural and urban unsignalized intersections.

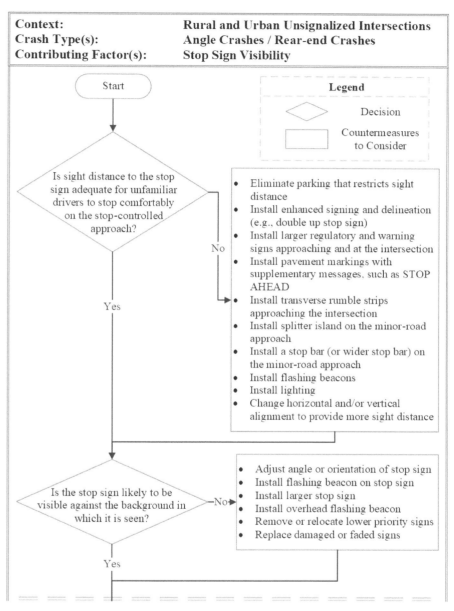

Figure 94.   Rural and urban unsignalized intersections; angle crashes, rear-end crashes; stop sign visibility.

(continued on next page)

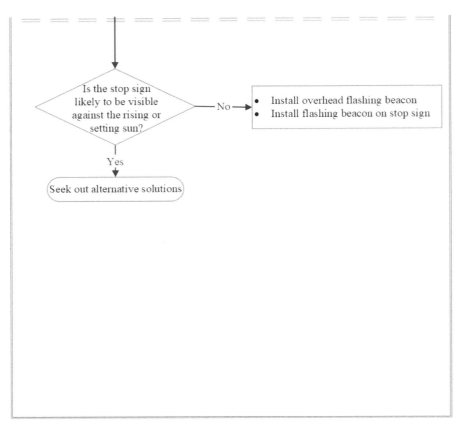

Figure 94. (Continued).

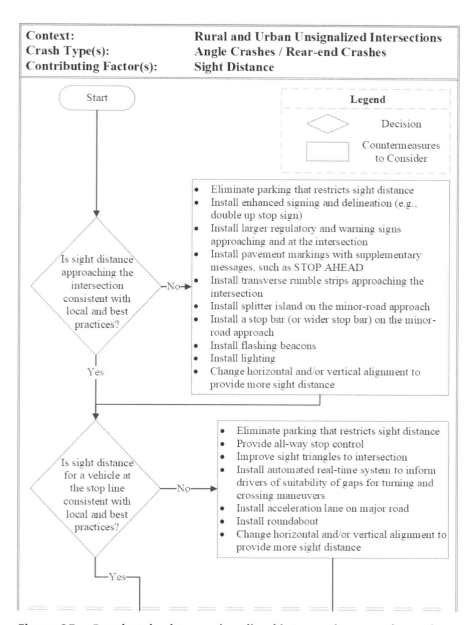

Context: Rural and Urban Unsignalized Intersections
Crash Type(s): Angle Crashes / Rear-end Crashes
Contributing Factor(s): Sight Distance

Start

Legend

◇ Decision

▭ Countermeasures to Consider

Is sight distance approaching the intersection consistent with local and best practices? —No→

- Eliminate parking that restricts sight distance
- Install enhanced signing and delineation (e.g., double up stop sign)
- Install larger regulatory and warning signs approaching and at the intersection
- Install pavement markings with supplementary messages, such as STOP AHEAD
- Install transverse rumble strips approaching the intersection
- Install splitter island on the minor-road approach
- Install a stop bar (or wider stop bar) on the minor-road approach
- Install flashing beacons
- Install lighting
- Change horizontal and/or vertical alignment to provide more sight distance

Yes

Is sight distance for a vehicle at the stop line consistent with local and best practices? —No→

- Eliminate parking that restricts sight distance
- Provide all-way stop control
- Improve sight triangles to intersection
- Install automated real-time system to inform drivers of suitability of gaps for turning and crossing maneuvers
- Install acceleration lane on major road
- Install roundabout
- Change horizontal and/or vertical alignment to provide more sight distance

Yes

Figure 95. Rural and urban unsignalized intersections; angle crashes, rear-end crashes; sight distance.

(continued on next page)

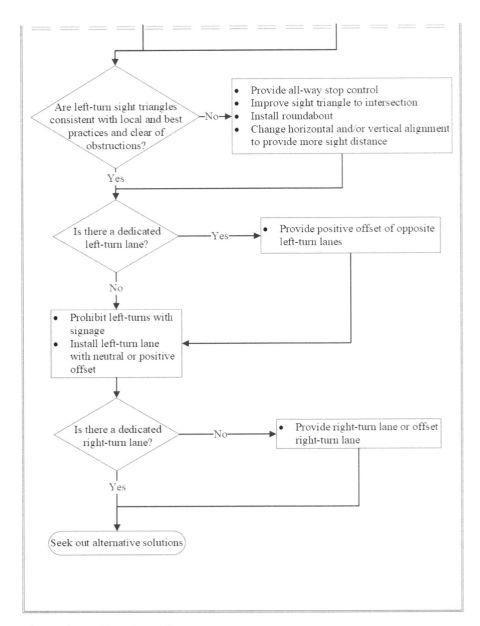

Figure 95. (Continued).

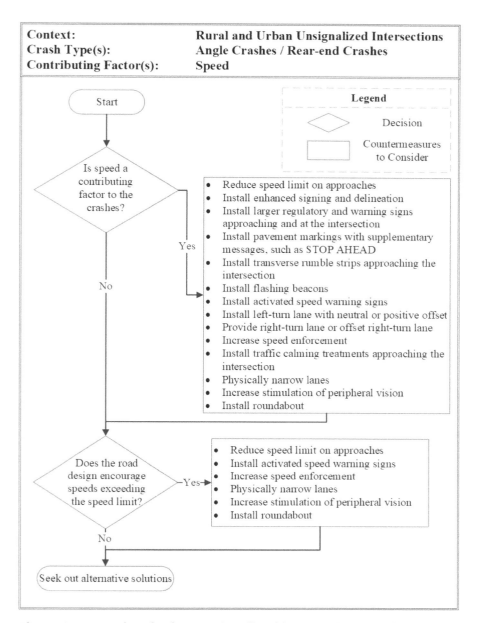

Figure 96. Rural and urban unsignalized intersections; angle crashes, rear-end crashes; speed.

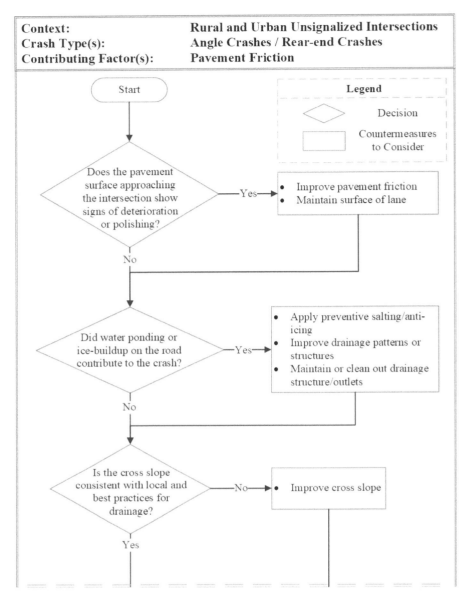

Figure 97.   Rural and urban unsignalized intersections; angle crashes, rear-end crashes; pavement friction.

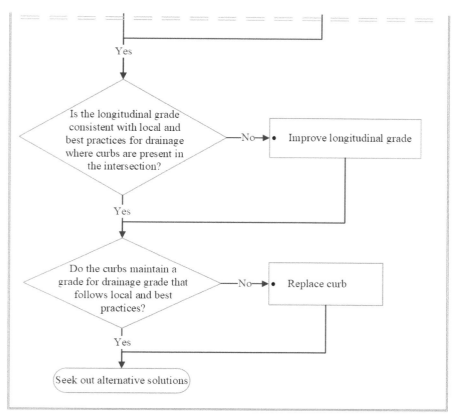

Figure 97.   (Continued).

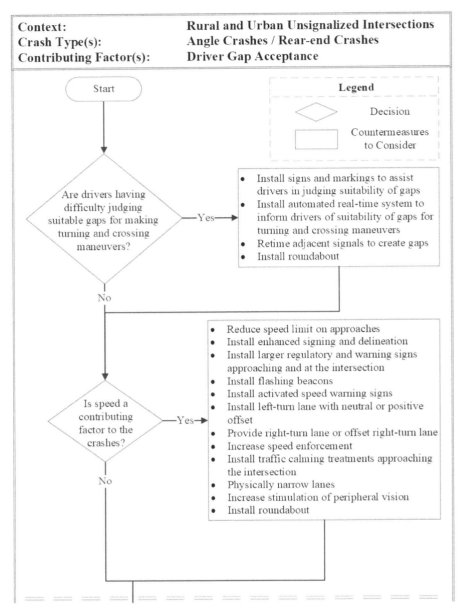

Figure 98.   Rural and urban unsignalized intersections; angle crashes, rear-end crashes; driver gap acceptance.

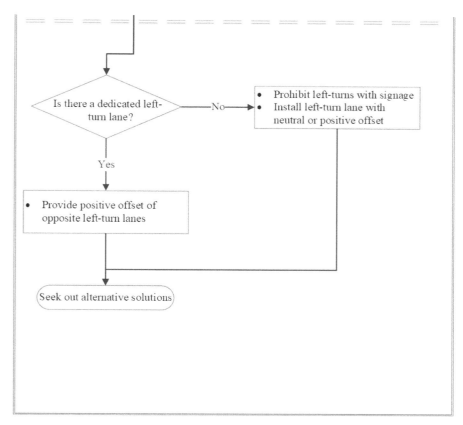

Figure 98.   (Continued).

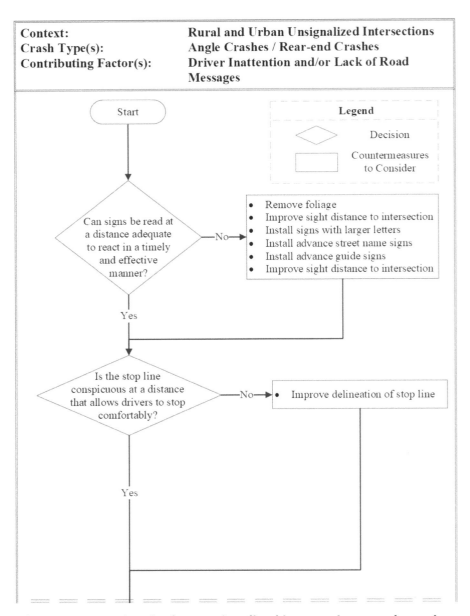

Figure 99. Rural and urban unsignalized intersections; angle crashes, rear-end crashes; driver inattention and/or lack of road messages.

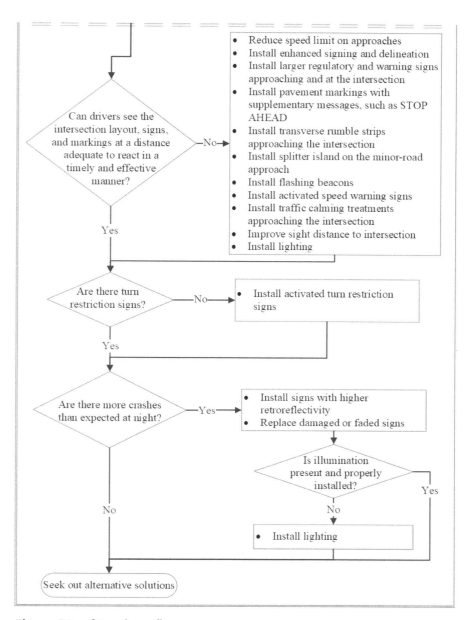

Figure 99. (Continued).

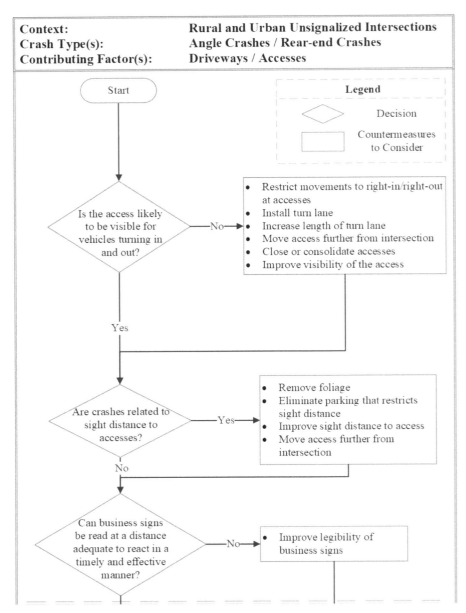

Figure 100.   Rural and urban unsignalized intersections; angle crashes, rear-end crashes; driveways/accesses.

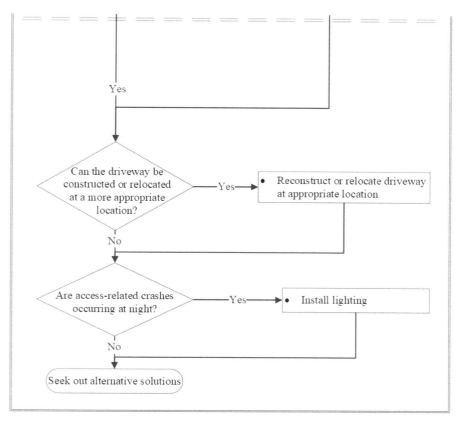

Figure 100.   (Continued).

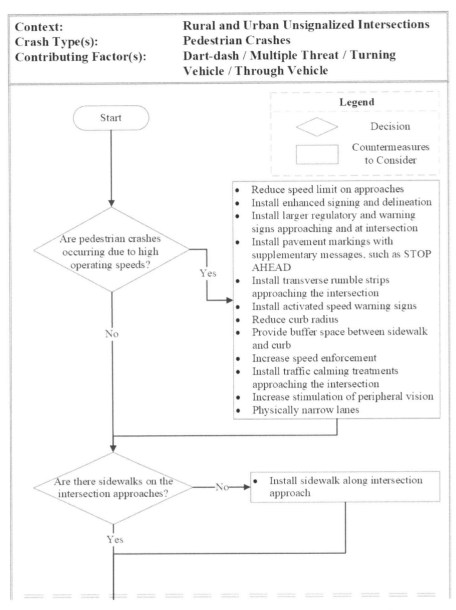

Figure 101.   Rural and urban unsignalized intersections; pedestrian crashes; dart-dash/multiple threat/turning vehicle/through vehicle.

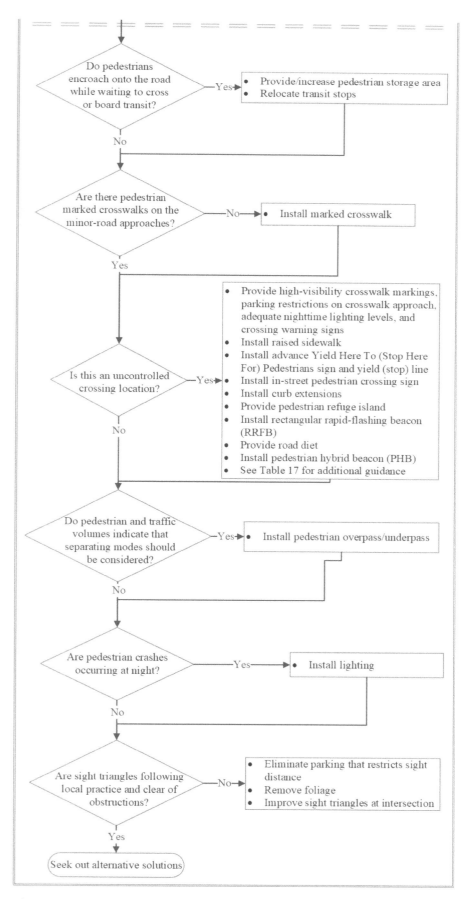

Figure 101. (Continued).

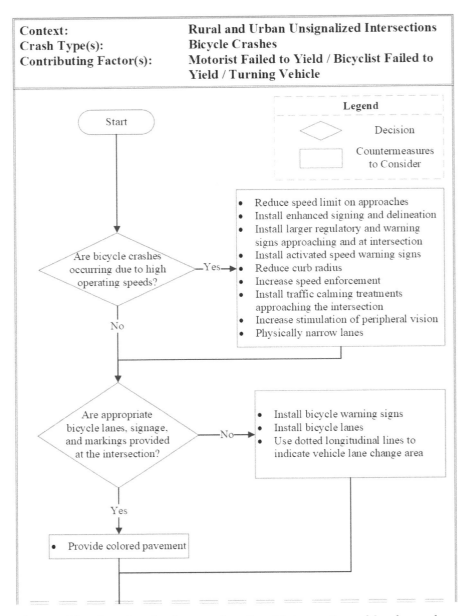

Figure 102.   Rural and urban unsignalized intersections; bicycle crashes; motorist failed to yield/bicyclist failed to yield/turning vehicle.

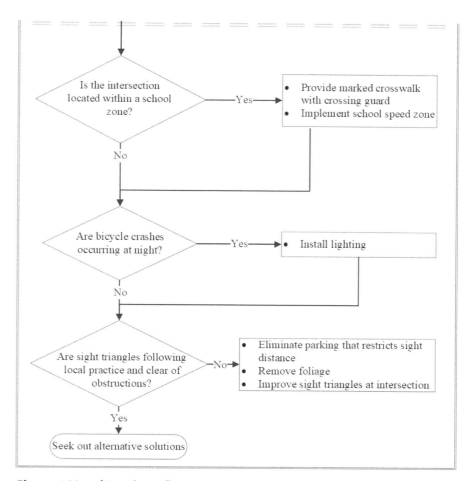

Figure 102.   (Continued).

CHAPTER 11

Procedures for Assessing Road User Demands

11.1 Quantifying Workload in Driving Tasks

Description. Practitioners can use this diagnostic method to identify the key elements of the driving task that shape the demands placed on the road user. This chapter provides step-by-step procedures for conducting workload analysis for a given roadway segment and driving task and shows how these methods can be adapted based on the scope and resources allocated toward this effort. Examples are provided to explain how to translate the results of these analyses into recommendations for revising roadway elements and traffic operations.

When to use: Driver errors occur because the demands of the driving task—the workload imposed on the drivers—exceed the driver's capabilities, especially when time is limited. As noted in Chapter 8, a useful shorthand for thinking about workload is to consider the time available to complete a task relative to the specific demands of the task; in other words, workload = time/task. Task analysis and workload assessment techniques can help practitioners answer basic questions about their roadway involving driver perception and behaviors (e.g., what is the roadway communicating to road users? How are drivers likely to respond?). The resulting information can help diagnose existing issues while reviewing environmental conditions, identifying crash patterns, and supporting countermeasure selection as part of the cost-benefit analysis of treatment or new design options. These techniques may also be used to support network screening and RSA activities. Both task analysis and workload assessment are established and well-documented techniques. Key data sources used to quantify workload-driving tasks include Richard et al. (2006), Tijerina et al. (1995b), Tignor (2022, 2023), and Messer (1980).

11.2 Introduction

The objective of this tool is to help practitioners assess roadway design and operations and to identify elements that impose a high demand on drivers. These methods aim to consider what a roadway requires of drivers and include at the very least the number of static and dynamic elements that require the driver's attention, comprehension, decisions, and potential action. The methods described in this tool are intended to help quantify the relative demand of the built environment. For example, the tool can be used to assess the differences between a minimally signed rural road with no access points versus one with multiple access points and extensive roadside signage; specific roadway contexts (e.g., illumination, geometry, and driver differences) can also be included in the analysis.

It is suggested that practitioners carefully read the material presented in sections 11.2.1 to 11.3 of this chapter because they provide the computational components that are used in the working example given in section 11.5 of this chapter.

11.2.1 What Is Workload?

Workload can be defined as the demands placed on an individual (e.g., drivers, pedestrians, bicyclists) by a particular activity, including effort, task complexity, time requirements, and the nature of possible interference between concurrent tasks (see Gartner and Murphy, 1979, Angell et al., 2006, and Gawron, 2000). Chapter 2: Human Factors of the HSM (AASHTO, 2010), discusses driver workload and human information processing limitations.

Workload is an internal construct—similar to attention—that describes the relationship between the demands of a task within an operating environment and the capabilities of the user or operator. In a roadway safety context, workload reflects the cumulative effect of specific demands imposed on the road user by the requirements of a specific task. These would include the demands placed on

- A driver as they approach an intersection or complex interchange,
- A pedestrian crossing a roadway, or
- A bicyclist riding on the shoulder or in a lane on a rural road.

For example, to complete their tasks, drivers, pedestrians, and bicyclists continuously perform several more granular subtasks at the same time, reflecting the multidimensional nature of travel. These tasks include

- Visually scanning the roadway environment,
- Identifying task-relevant elements (e.g., other road users, vehicles, geometric elements, traffic signs, and traffic signals),
- Maintaining position in a driving lane or a sidewalk, and
- Controlling speed.

Critically, the travel environment is ever-changing, and responsive road users allocate relatively high levels of vigilance and attention to these tasks.

What are some specific examples of these demands? As summarized in Chapter 8, typically the combined effects of three key types of demands are considered: perceptual (e.g., detecting and making sense of what drivers see, hear, and feel), decision-making/cognitive (e.g., integrating what you perceive with things you know, such as rules-of-the-road or your previous experience with a roadway facility to decide what to do), and psychomotor/response (e.g., executing a decision-taking action, that is, changing your gaze to somewhere else within the visual scene, braking, or changing lanes) (Richard et al., 2006).

11.2.2 Workload and Driving Performance

Performance can be impacted whenever there is a mismatch between task/environmental demands and road user capabilities, that is, if workload is too high or too low (see Chapter 8). Generally, though, the issues arise when workload is too high; driver overload is a significant contributor to driver errors and subsequent road safety (Singh, 2015). Road user performance errors might include the following:

- Failure to perceive conditions because of distraction and/or inattention
- Incorrect assumptions about appropriate behaviors
- Failure to respond to demands or hazards in an appropriate and/or timely fashion
- Incorrect action (see also Wierwille et al., 2002)

For drivers, a low workload may increase fatigue, and drivers who are already fatigued may exhibit errors under a high workload because fatigue reduces a driver's available resources (cognitive resources) (Matthews and Reinerman-Jones, 2017). Determining measures of driver workload is important to reduce driver error and plan, design, and operate road systems that can tolerate driver error (see Chapter 3: Diagnostic Assessment in the Safe System).

Workload is a challenge to measure, in part because it reflects characteristics inherent to the individual being measured—such as experience, ability, age, and so forth—but also because it depends on task- and environment-specific infrastructure elements that influence task demand and difficulty. Specifically, measuring workload requires an activity to quantify; thus, task analysis and workload measurement go hand-in-hand.

Three different approaches to measuring workload that vary in terms of their complexity and focus are discussed in this chapter. There are relatively few studies that have examined workload in the roadway context, and those studies have focused on driver workload. Thus, much of the discussion focuses on drivers and driver activities. However, the same general principles and procedures used to assess workload for drivers can be used to assess workload for pedestrians and bicyclists.

As discussed in Chapter 8, task and workload analyses are routinely conducted during the development and design of many human-machine systems, especially military systems. In this regard, a favored approach to assessing workload that has been used in the past in the aviation domain is the Task Analysis/Workload (TAWL) technique (Hamilton et al., 1991). It is especially useful for assessing and analyzing workload in situations where other measures of workload (e.g., direct measures of performance or subjective measures from actual users) are unavailable or otherwise impractical to obtain. Some key benefits of the TAWL approach are that it connects workload estimates to the mental and physical requirements of specific tasks associated with the activity. Thus, the approach supports the identification of design alternatives that could lower workload.

Originally developed to assess workload for helicopter pilots, the TAWL technique involves the successive decomposition of a scenario (e.g., making a left turn at a signalized intersection) into segments, tasks, and subtasks, with specific information processing requirements and workload estimates developed at the subtask level. Critically, the application of these techniques requires no formal training in psychology, human factors, or the measurement or analysis of workload. This approach has been used to conduct workload analyses for the FHWA (Richard et al., 2006) and is discussed below as the Direct Driver Measurement, Task Analysis, and Relative Workload approach (see section 11.3 of this chapter).

However, the decomposition of tasks into subtasks does not directly provide information about the relative demands of the driving task that can impact driving performance. Three key task elements relating to the context of a specific roadway are relevant to measuring and analyzing workload:

Task Time: In the driving context, many tasks are time-limited based on speed, with greater speeds translating into reduced task time. Generally, more difficult tasks take more time to complete, and generally, reduced time to complete tasks translates into a higher workload with possible impacts on driver performance and safety. Road users can make trade-offs between task time and accuracy (e.g., a driver coming to a full stop at a stop sign) (Angell et al., 2006). Related to this is the "time window" a user has to complete a task. Within the time window, tasks can be

- Forced-paced, where task timing and execution are mostly determined by factors outside of the driver's control, or
- Self-paced, where the driver is mostly in control of task timing and execution (Richard et al., 2006).

In the case of a driver making a left turn across the path, the driver's task includes finding an acceptable gap in the opposing traffic and then turning. This task is forced paced if the driver is forced to act within a tightly prescribed time window (e.g., making a left turn across traffic as the traffic signal changes from yellow to red). On the other hand, this task is a self-paced task if the driver has more control over the timing of the task (e.g., making a left turn across traffic at an uncontrolled intersection).

Task Concurrency: Road users have a finite pool of mental resources (see Chapter 2) that can be applied to the travel tasks at hand such as catching a bus, driving on an urban street, or riding a bicycle along a trail. In general, a higher workload is associated with multiple demands that compete for the same mental resources (e.g., multiple signs on both sides of the street at the same location competing for the driver's visual attention). Interference between concurrent tasks reflects basic human limitations; for example: (1) drivers cannot look at two separate locations in the visual field simultaneously and (2) their ability to attend to navigation instructions while carrying on a conversation is degraded. Concurrent tasks that draw from the same mental resources can interfere with operator performance on one or both tasks. This understanding of flexible but finite mental resources helps explain how challenging single-tasks (e.g., making a left turn across traffic) can run into processing issues and how dual-task performance is more likely to be hampered by simultaneously performing similar tasks (e.g., looking at and manually tuning a radio while driving) than by simultaneously performing dissimilar tasks (e.g., merely listening to the radio while driving).

Individual Differences: Driver populations may experience different levels of workload along a similar stretch of roadway because of their capabilities, expectations, and driving skills. Consider an older driver with reduced perceptual capabilities (e.g., degraded night vision) or reduced physical capabilities (e.g., slower braking response); certain situations might place higher demands on that older driver, leading to a higher workload relative to a younger driver. Other factors, such as driving skill and familiarity, also play a role; a highly skilled driver may experience less workload compared to a less-skilled driver when navigating a particular section of roadway for the first time. Individual differences (e.g., for the older road user) will often have unique performance implications based on transportation modality (e.g., older driver, older pedestrian, older cyclist).

11.3 Methods for Assessing Driver Workload

Practitioners can answer basic driver perception and behavior questions about their roadway using TAWL techniques (e.g., what is the roadway communicating to road users?). How are drivers likely to respond to specific driving requirements? The resulting information can help diagnose existing issues while identifying crash patterns and supporting countermeasure selection as part of the cost-benefit analysis of treatment or new design options. These techniques may also be used to support network screening and RSA activities.

For example, in Figure 103, two roadway designs are being compared during a planning effort. Option A, with a quarter-mile signal spacing, and Option B, with half-mile signal spacing with access control, may be compared based on travel time and travel delay spacings, but they can also be evaluated based on roadway demands. For example, Option B reduces conflict points (i.e., points of potential collision where vehicle paths overlap) and creates greater spacing between conflict areas which helps simplify the driving task and reduces driver workload and travel time.

Figure 104 outlines a sequence of steps that can be used to select a workload measurement method and conduct a workload analysis. There are several options for measuring and modeling workload (see reviews by Gawron, 2000; Matthews and Reinerman-Jones, 2017), and in general, for conducting task analyses. This tool describes three approaches, each with their respective strengths and limitations (see Table 18) and the level of information they incorporate into the workload assessment (see Table 19).

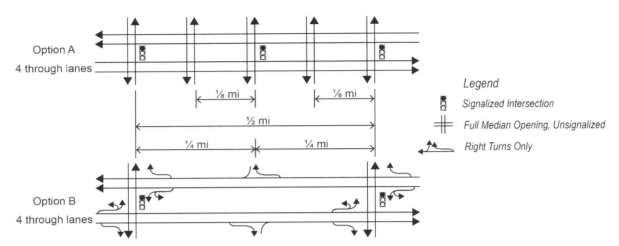

Figure 103.   During a planning effort, roadway design options such as Option A and Option B may be evaluated and compared based on roadway demand (Source: Williams et al., 2014).

Two of these methods (Approaches 1 and 3) use a hierarchical-task analysis as the basis for the workload analysis (Stuster, 2019). The more robust, empirical approach, Direct Driver Measurement, Task Analysis, and Relative Workload, defines the roadway tasks and associated workload based on actual observations of real tasks completed by real drivers and identifies key "information bottlenecks" and locations and activities where roadway demands can exceed the capabilities of road users (sections 11.3.1, 11.3.2, and 11.3.9 of this chapter). The second approach, Analytical Inventory of Demands based on Roadway Features, enables the practitioner to generate estimates indicating where high roadway demands exist as a proxy for driver overload (sections 11.3.1, 11.3.3, 11.3.4, and 11.3.9). It involves examining the location of roadway elements relative to each other and to the tasks drivers are expected to perform to provide insight into locations or elements that might expose them to roadway demands that they are unable to meet without experiencing degraded task performance (section 11.3.4 of this chapter). The third approach, Analytical Task Analysis and Relative Workload, also identifies information bottlenecks, but rather than requiring empirical data from actual drivers, the practitioner bases their roadway assessment on existing data (perhaps from previously published task/workload analyses), virtual or real drive-throughs on a particular facility, and their own experience (sections 11.3.1, 11.3.3, and 11.3.5 to 11.3.9). Thus Approach 3 replaces empirical data obtained from actual drivers in Approach 1 with some form of expert judgement. The second approach may be completed relatively quickly compared to the first and third approaches, but it may not capture how drivers interact with specific roadway features and may not account for cumulative demands. Specifically, a particular stretch of roadway could be deemed to be high workload using these techniques because it might have many driveways, even though most are highly visible and known to be lightly traveled. Conversely, even a freeway interchange can truly be a high workload if it lacks infrastructure support, such as signs and markings. In short, caution is advised—while counts of key infrastructure elements are an indicator of possible demand, they may not always equate to a higher workload.

11.3.1 Collect Roadway Section Data

Perform a walk-through for the roadway of interest, and document potential hazards (e.g., conflict points), information sources (e.g., signs, traffic control devices), and road characteristics (e.g., horizontal curves, grades, bridges, roadside hardware) along the route. When evaluating

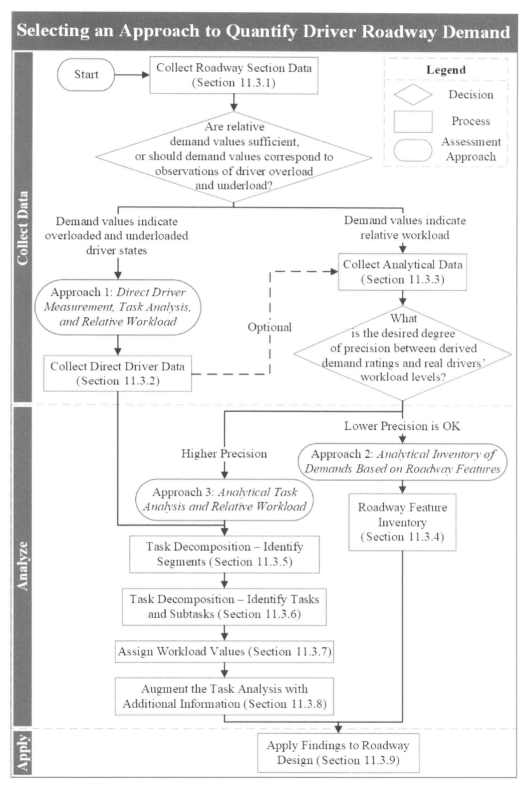

Figure 104.   An outline of steps to follow for each workload assessment approach.

Table 18.   An overview of strengths and limitations of each of the three approaches presented in this toolkit for measuring workload.

Strengths, Limitations, and Examples	Approach 1: Direct Driver Measurement, Task Analysis, and Relative Workload	Approach 2: Analytical Inventory of Demands Based on Roadway Features	Approach 3: Analytical Task Analysis and Relative Workload
Strengths	• Collects more precise real-time measures of workload • Uses empirical data from drivers • May observe tasks or coping strategies that are repeated between drivers relevant to the specific roadway but may not have been identified during analytical activities • If recruiting from diverse populations (e.g., familiar versus unfamiliar drivers, older drivers), practitioners may observe variations between groups that are useful for design considerations	• A relatively quick procedure based on roadway feature counts, exposure times, and traffic flow	• Replaces empirical data from actual drivers with expert judgement • Option to include visual demands and information sources • Option to include data/evidence from the literature regarding the expected performance • Option to identify information processing bottlenecks—key locations, activities where roadway demands can exceed the capabilities of road users • Uniquely suited to identifying high-workload and time-constrained activities and roadway locations
Limitations	• Requires more time and effort to collect and analyze the data	• The procedure can quantify relative demands imposed by different roadway design options as a proxy for workload, but there are cases where the driver's workload will not correlate to the number of features.	• Some task decomposition determinations require expert judgment • May not capture individual differences across a group of actual drivers
Examples	Stuster and Roesch, 2001 Shafer, 1996	Tignor, 2022, 2023 Habib et al., 2019	Richard et al., 2006 Richard and Lichty, 2013 Hamilton et al., 1991

Table 19.   Key tasks elements that can be obtained through each of the three approaches presented in this toolset.

	Individual differences and capabilities	Concurrent tasks and competing demands	Time
Direct Driver Measurement, Task Analysis, and Relative Workload (Approach 1)	●	●	●
Analytical Inventory of Demands based on Roadway Features (Approach 2)		○	●
Analytical Task Analysis and Relative Workload (Approach 3)		●	●

Note: ○ Tool Provides Partial Information

● Tool Provides Significant Information

Blank cells indicate the tool provides little or no information for the respective category.

existing roads, useful data can be gathered by driving the roadway in both directions while recording forward video on a dashboard camera. When evaluating roads that have not yet been implemented (e.g., during a planning activity), practitioners may identify key roadway characteristics from drawings, area photographs, MUTCD design requirements, and videos of roadways with similar facilities. Analytical tools used by the practitioners to collect roadway section data include route maps, existing task analyses for generic road designs, videos, drone footage, internet-based mapping applications (e.g., Google Maps), and photographs.

This is a key step in determining which of the three approaches to measuring workload will be required. As indicated in Figure 104, once these basic data have been obtained, the analyst should determine if relative workload/demand values are sufficient (i.e., Approaches 2 or 3), or if more precise estimates of driver workload are needed (i.e., Approach 1).

11.3.2 Collect Direct Driver Data

Obtaining workload measures directly from drivers is the key distinction between Approach 1 and Approach 3. In Approach 1, the most direct way to identify driving tasks is by observing real drivers driving through a facility and obtaining workload data directly from them based on what they do. Although it requires time and resources to collect such data, the value of this activity is that the practitioner can build a task structure based on real driving tasks, collect objective or subjective data on demand imposed in the specific driving context, and collect information that reflects individual differences across drivers. Direct data collection for workload can be performed on small groups of drivers [e.g., Tijerina et al. (1995b) observed seven drivers in a pilot study and 37 drivers in a follow-up study (Tijerina et al., 1996) where they could account for individual differences]. This analysis also allows the practitioners to observe individual differences between driver groups of interest (e.g., familiar versus unfamiliar drivers and older versus younger drivers) that may be useful for design considerations.

- For example, a specific roadway sign can impose a demand on the driver that depends on the moment-to-moment requirements of the task and
  - The sign's meaning to the driver,
  - Driver expectancy,
  - Driver experience,
  - Driver familiarity with the roadway and road segments, and
  - Individual differences in performance capabilities.

The most straightforward option for direct data collection is to use dashboard-mounted cameras to record roadway-facing and driver-facing videos. These videos may be analyzed to identify specific actions drivers take, when drivers are taking those actions, and the general location of visual data sampled by the drivers before those actions. Common tasks and themes may be compared across drivers to form the basis of the task analysis.

As part of this data collection effort, several optional methods exist to measure and model workload (Gawron, 2000; Matthews and Reinerman-Jones, 2017). For example, an eye tracker may provide more granular information about visual cues sampled by drivers, requesting drivers to respond to subjective workload scales after driving or after roadway segments of interest. Similar efforts use the Cooper-Harper Scale (Fitzpatrick et al., 2000) and NASA Task-Load Index (TLX) (Xie et al., 2019). For practitioners with access to the appropriate equipment, collecting data from participants using occlusion goggles in the presence of a safety driver can provide real-time measures of workload based on how frequently participants request visual information via a foot pedal on the floor of the vehicle (Shafer, 1996). Analytical tools used by the practitioners to collect direct driver data include videos, surveys, eye trackers (optional), and occlusion goggles (optional).

11.3.3 Collect Analytical Data

In the absence or as an accompaniment to original data collection, the practitioner can collect data about relevant driving tasks using alternative data sources, including existing literature that describes relevant task analyses and other data sources describing how drivers are expected to complete certain maneuvers to be an attentive driver or what kind of information they may encounter within specific-roadway environments (e.g., state driver manuals, MUTCD). Practitioners may also facilitate task identification by recording driver-facing videos of themselves or project team members driving through a facility. However, a single driver video may be useful to identify tasks, but these observations may not apply to the broader driving population. Analytical tools used by the practitioners to collect analytical data include videos, state driver guides, MUTCD, and existing task analyses.

11.3.4 Roadway Feature Inventory

As noted earlier, the second approach, Analytical Inventory of Demands based on Roadway Features, enables the practitioner to generate estimates indicating where strong roadway demands exist as a proxy for a more driver-based workload assessment. This approach involves examining the location and measurable characteristics of static and dynamic roadway features. Similar to identifying roadway segments, here, the practitioner divides the segment of interest into clusters and non-clusters (i.e., roadway segments between clusters) based on their determination that the geometric and traffic conditions within the clusters are qualitatively different, based on relative counts of the static and dynamic elements, along with exposure time within segments. Static and dynamic feature metrics are examined between all segments of interest (i.e., clusters and non-clusters) to provide insight into locations or elements that might expose them to roadway demands that they are unable to meet without experiencing degraded task performance. This approach may be completed relatively quickly, but it may not capture how drivers interact with specific roadway features and may not account for cumulative demands. Data gathered during the diagnostic process may be augmented with lidar, drone footage, and GPS data, especially for analyzing horizontal and vertical curve parameters (e.g., Habib et al., 2019; Tignor, 2022, 2023).

In this step, the practitioner quantifies the demands placed on road users by the presence of infrastructure elements relative to cluster traversal time and renewal time (i.e., time between clusters). Potential metrics to collect are

- The number of geometric features (e.g., channelized intersections and railroad grade crossings) (Messer, 1980; Habib et al., 2019);
- The time between driveways, curves, and tangents;
- Time spacing of warning and regulatory signs by direction;
- Percent grades and grade travel time;
- Percent next to the guardrail and rock fences;
- Percent horizontal curve and travel time (Tignor, 2022, 2023); and
- The number of conflict and access points (the number and type of conflict points impact safety) (FHWA, 2022c).

These individual metrics may be tabulated and compared between roadway segments or proposed designs. In addition, several ways are proposed in the literature to create aggregate metrics based on pre-determined demand ratings by geometric feature tables (Messer, 1980) or for derived demand ratings (Tignor, 2022, 2023).

While roadway feature inventory approaches are helpful because they explicitly link driver workload to static and dynamic infrastructure features—especially geometric features—they focus on macro features of the infrastructure; they lack, in exchange for simplicity, a detailed assessment of the specific demands that are placed on the driver by a conjoint set of driving demands for a particular driving maneuver. For example, these approaches do not consider perceptual, cognitive, and psychomotor demands in a time-sequenced manner that would more precisely identify roadway sections with high workload. Thus, a particular stretch of roadway could be deemed high workload through these techniques because it might have many driveways, even though most are highly visible and known to be lightly traveled. Conversely, even a freeway interchange can truly be a high workload if it lacks infrastructure support, such as signs or markings. That is, an increase in infrastructure elements may or may not equate to a higher workload. Simplified approaches may or may not provide diagnostic information that can identify effective countermeasures when the workload is too high. Analytical tools used by practitioners to quantify roadway feature demands include generated roadway segments, optional lidar and GPS data, and workload rating lookup tables (Messer, 1980; Tignor, 2022, 2023).

11.3.5 Task Decomposition–Identify Segments

The roadway being evaluated may be divided into a series of time- or location-based segments, usually three to six per roadway of interest (Richard et al., 2006). Segments generally represent a related set of driving tasks geared toward a common goal or driving objective (e.g., decelerating or executing a turn). Changes in roadway speed may also be used to define segments since changes in driver speed affect time constraints and the rate of information presented from the roadway environment (Richard et al., 2006).

11.3.6 Task Decomposition–Identify Tasks and Subtasks

Driving tasks may be decomposed into successively smaller activities to characterize what a driver does and how they do it. The tasks represent information that needs to be obtained, decisions that need to be made, and actions that need to be taken during a particular roadway segment. The objective of this task decomposition is to identify the relative amounts of workload within a task and the nature of the workload and to establish when drivers might experience workload peaks that could lead to a reduction in driving performance. Task decomposition may be applied to standard roadway designs as well as roadway segments or locations that have unique designs or operational issues.

Task decomposition stops when the tasks and subtasks are decomposed into information processing elements (e.g., perceptual, cognitive, and psychomotor).

Perceptual subtasks involve sensing (e.g., seeing, hearing, smelling, and feeling, as the most common driving task senses) stimuli from the environment, which can range from the simple detection of brake lights to visually inspecting a gauge status to actively searching for a roadway guide sign.

Cognitive subtasks involve decisions and judgments where a driver processes, interprets, or evaluates information they possess to complete a task. Relevant activities can range from basic decisions, like emergency braking, to judging the distance until an upcoming stop sign to judging the distance and speed of oncoming vehicles when making a left turn.

Psychomotor subtasks involve physical actions, such as making simple adjustments to the steering wheel to maintain lane position on a straight road or manually turning a radio dial to find a station, to more complex actions such as the coordinated movements used to change gears when operating a manual transmission. Head and eye movements that support and quantify eye glances are not included since this level of granularity reduces the practicality and efficiency of this method.

Although not all tasks or subtasks identified in the task decomposition will be performed exhaustively by all drivers, these lists indicate reasonable sets of tasks drivers are likely to perform to successfully navigate a section of roadway.

11.3.7 Assign Workload Values

As shown in Table 20, within each task, workload values for subtasks can be assigned based on a workload estimation tool for perceptual, cognitive, and psychomotor information processing demands in driving described in a previous FHWA report (Richard et al., 2006). The total perceptual, cognitive, and psychomotor workload values are summed for each task. These total values were used to estimate the workload that tasks imposed on the drivers during each segment on the roadway of interest. Analytical tools used by practitioners for assigned workload values

Table 20. Workload estimation tool from Richard et al. (2006).

Estimate (Perceptual)	Definition (Perceptual)	Example (Perceptual)
1	Register or detect visual or auditory stimulus; detect motion	Detect brake lights or onset of headlights and register vehicle heading and relative speed. Hear siren.
2	Discriminate differences in visual or auditory stimuli	Determine traffic signal status. Determine if a sound is car horn or siren.
3	Visually inspect general viewing/check or listen to sound	Check fuel gauge status. Listen to music. View roadway feature.
4	Visually locate/align or orient to sound	Determine position of a roadway object or feature. Determine the location from where a siren is coming.
5	Visually track/follow or monitor	Track a potential hazard (e.g., cyclist approaching on cross street). Monitor the position of a moving vehicle.
6	Visually read (symbol)	Read an unfamiliar street sign.
7	Visually scan/search or find object	Search for hazards. Search for street signs.
Estimate (Cognitive)	**Definition (Cognitive)**	**Example (Cognitive)**
1	Simple, automatic response	Perform emergency braking. Maintain lane. Respond automatically or with conditioned responses (shoulder check during lane change).
2	Alternative selection	Decide response. Is traffic signal green? Is a vehicle stopped?
3	Sign/signal recognition	Recognize street sign or familiar intersection or roadway furniture. Determine if-then relationships.
4	Evaluation/judgment of single aspect	Judge distance to intersection. Determine whether a decelerating vehicle is stopping/time estimation.
5	Encoding/decoding, recall	Remember instructions or an address. Interpret an unfamiliar traffic sign. Extrapolate posted traffic rules into allowable driving actions.
6	Evaluation/judgment of several aspects	Judge the safe gap sizes given speed, distance, and traction of oncoming traffic.
7	Estimation, calculation, conversion	Convert miles into kilometers.
Estimate (Psychomotor)	**Definition (Psychomotor)**	**Example (Psychomotor)**
1	Simple, feedback controlled, automatic responses	Make steering wheel adjustments for lane maintenance. Head/eye movements.
2	Discrete actuation	Depress button. Activate signal. Perform emergency braking.
3	Continuous adjustment	Change extent to which the accelerator is depressed to change speed. Turn steering wheel through a turn.
4	Manipulative	Tune digital radio.
5	Symbolic production	Write down instructions.
6	Serial discrete manipulation	Dial phone number. Use telematics system.
7	Temporally coordinated unlearned serial actions	Learning to drive a manual transmission.

include generated subtasks and workload-rating lookup tables (Richard et al., 2006). If Approach 1 is being used, the drivers can provide these workload values during or after the test drives.

11.3.8 Augment the Task Analysis with Additional Information

To create the graphical workload estimation profiles, tasks and subtasks are characterized by temporal limitations and constraints (e.g., time windows, self- versus forced-paced activities, concurrent tasks). In practice, scenario segments may be divided into four to six time intervals representing different periods when each task can occur. The tasks are then arranged into intervals based on the logical precedence of the tasks and whether individual tasks may occur concurrently (similar to the approach seen in Richard et al., 2006). The workload estimates from all tasks within each interval are summed to create the workload profiles. When tasks are self-paced rather than forced-paced, the workload for the task is only summed into the initial segment time interval where the driver could complete it. The purpose of this method is to identify intervals within each scenario where demands placed on the driver are higher relative to other intervals instead of drawing conclusions about driver performance or vehicle safety from the workload values. The rationale is that it will be more difficult for drivers to cope with driving demands during intervals where they attempt more tasks or tasks with a higher difficulty level than during intervals with fewer or easier tasks (Richard et al., 2006). Thus, the workload profiles depict where multiple factors (e.g., forced-paced tasks and high workload) may converge to create potential information processing bottlenecks (Richard et al., 2006).

11.3.9 Apply Findings to Roadway Design

The purpose of these methods is to help support driver safety and performance through facility design. In their implementation of Approach 2: Analytical Inventory of Demands based on Roadway Features, Habib et al. (2019) found that their Workload Index ratings were correlated to observed collision rates on the roadways of interest: for every one-unit increment on the Workload Index, the collision rate increased by 7.1%. A practical application of the information derived from these methods would be to identify (1) locations where complex signage could create roadway demand peaks and (2) locations where signage would support timely driver perception and interpretation of task-relevant information.

The three methods described in this toolset can help place workload in the context of task demands, where task demands refer to the requirements that the facility or roadway segment or a maneuver within the facility or roadway segment places on a road user in terms of perceiving and interpreting the environment, making decisions, and then executing those decisions. Furthermore, Approach 1: Direct Driver Measurement, Task Analysis, and Relative Workload and Approach 3: Analytical Task Analysis and Relative Workload allow for a comparison of task demands to the capabilities of the driver. Using Approach 1, the practitioner may observe real drivers and identify instances of driver overload and underload through direct observational data (e.g., video, eye tracking), subjective data obtained from the drivers (e.g., NASA TLX), or through changes in driving performance (Gawron, 2000; Matthews and Reinerman-Jones, 2017). The practitioner can also determine aspects of demand shaped by

- Driver expectancy,
- Driver experience,
- Driver familiarity with the roadway, and
- Individual differences in performance capabilities.

Approach 2: Analytical Inventory of Demands based on Roadway Features provides a simplified method of estimating workload by road segments.

All three approaches allow the practitioner, with varying levels of precision, to quantify relative demands that drivers are expected to cope with while driving through a facility and identify parts of the roadway where multiple factors (e.g., forced-paced tasks and high workload) may converge to create potential information processing bottlenecks (Richard et al., 2006). A key limitation of these approaches is that conducting effective workload analyses benefits from some applied experience. However, at a basic level, the purpose of these approaches is to provide practitioners with ways to think about, question, and identify design choices that could place excessive demands on drivers traversing a facility. The outcomes of these methods can serve to help the practitioner consider or address the following questions:

- From the crashes/conflicts observed, do there seem to be any patterns that would indicate that workload was a contributing factor? Are there any discernible patterns between or among PDO crashes and conflicts compared to crashes and conflicts involving serious injuries or fatal crashes?
- What features may impose workload (e.g., signs, traffic signals, dynamic movement of vehicles and pedestrians, watching for hazards, or changing geometric features)?
- Where are potential conflict points and how many are there?
- What expectations may drivers form based on how information is communicated throughout the facility? Can these expectations lead to unintended driver behaviors?
- Within the facility, are there any possible sources of confusion for a road user trying to extract information from the road geometry, infrastructure, and traffic control information? Specifically, is there consistency and meaning, or a lack thereof, to the geometrics, signs, markings, and traffic control devices that road users rely on?
- Taking into consideration user tasks and subsequent workload demands, are there any activities that suggest the presence of information processing bottlenecks (i.e., competing concurrent roadway demands that might cause task interference or unduly increase perceptual, cognitive, or psychomotor requirements for the road user)?
- Are there any unique environmental or road conditions that substantially increase road user stress, provide insufficient time for the road user to perceive and extract roadway information, or respond to hazards at conflict points (e.g., short acceleration/deceleration lanes, unexpected placement of roadside hardware, unexpected quickly narrowed lane widths, significant visibility restrictions, steep grades, and so forth)?
- What design or operational changes could help manage workload or align design intention with driver expectations? Could drivers be provided with more time to perceive and react appropriately to roadway information? Can these issues be mitigated by changes to geometry, signage, and/or traffic operations?

11.4 Working Example of Approach 2: Analytical Inventory of Demands based on Roadway Features

The following example is a short application of Approach 2: Analytical Inventory of Demands based on Roadway Features. This approach usually breaks up a roadway segment into clusters and non-clusters that have geometric and traffic conditions that are inherently different from one another. To support the comparison of the driver workload assessment approaches within this toolset, the following example applies Approach 2 to the same roadway and roadway segments used in the working example for Approach 3 (section 11.5 of this chapter). In addition, Approach 2 can document both dynamic and static roadway features, but this example focuses on static roadway features. Practitioners may refer to Tignor (2022, 2023) for thorough step-by-step demonstrations of Approach 2. This example breaks down the steps used to characterize and evaluate the relative workload of a driver traveling northeast on a curve located on Sand Point Way NE in Seattle, WA.

- **Step 1:** Collect roadway section data (Tool: section 11.3.1)
- **Step 2:** Roadway feature inventory (Tool: section 11.3.4)
- **Step 3:** Quantify roadway feature demands (Tool: section 11.3.4)

Table 21.   The documented route information after the collect roadway section data step is complete includes a schematic of the roadway of interest.

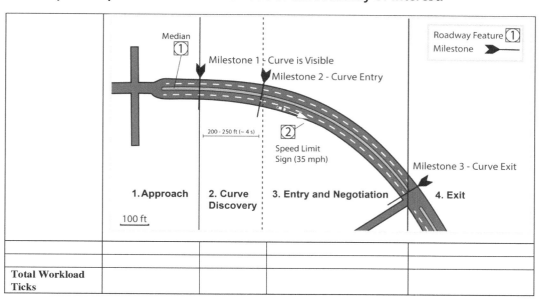

Total Workload Ticks				

In Step 1, the roadway is characterized and documented using route maps, photographs, drone footage, and videos collected by the practitioner. Static elements of interest (e.g., curve entry, regulatory signs, and intersections) are identified, and their locations are documented (Table 21). Usually, the practitioner would break up the roadway of interest into clusters and non-clusters that have geometric and traffic conditions that are inherently different from one another; however, in this case, the roadway has been divided into the clusters based on the roadway segments used in the Approach 3 working example. In this example, Segment 1: Approach starts after the left-most intersection (Table 21).

In Step 2, the static elements of interest are quantified and the number of static roadway features of interest within the clusters is identified (Table 22).

In Step 3, additional metrics are derived from the roadway feature counts to normalize these data based on cluster distance or traversal time. Then the individual metrics are tabulated and compared between clusters. In each metric row, the "most" demanding workload values are bolded and counted as one workload "tick." The total number of ticks in each segment column is summed to provide a measure of the relative demand exerted on the road user by the roadway features and infrastructure (Table 23).

11.5 Working Example of Approach 3: Quantifying the Demands and Relative Workload for a Heavy Truck Driver Traversing Around a Curve

The following example is a specific, but partial application of Approach 3: Analytical Task Analysis and Relative Workload and demonstrates how a practitioner could apply the general methods and tools described in sections 11.3.1, 11.3.3, and 11.3.5 through 11.3.8 of this chapter. This example breaks down the steps used to characterize and evaluate the relative workload of heavy truck drivers traversing a curve in normal driving conditions. Note that the example does not include dynamic roadway features. However, dynamic roadway features should be

Table 22.   The documented route information after the roadway feature inventory step is complete includes the initial metrics associated with the roadway's features of interest.

	1. Approach	2. Curve Discovery	3. Entry and Negotiation	4. Exit
Travel distance (ft)	100	250	700	200
Speed limit (mph)	35	35	35	35
Lane width (ft)	10	10	11	11
Shoulder width (ft)	4	4	3	5
Driveway frequency (#; #/mi)	1;	4;	1;	0;
Regulatory signs (#)	0	1	7	2
Warning signs (#)	0	0	0	1
% horizontal curve	0	0	100%	0
% grade	2%	2.8%	2.3%	0%
Unsignalized intersections	0	0	0	1
Bus stops	0	1	0	0
Total Workload Ticks				

included in the task and workload analysis if they are likely to be experienced by a typical driver while driving the facility under study.

- **Step 1:** Collect roadway section data (Tool: section 11.3.1; Example: section 11.5.1)
- **Step 2:** Collect analytical data (Tool: section 11.3.3; Example: section 11.5.2)
- **Step 3:** Task decomposition–identify segments (Tool: section 11.3.5; Example: section 11.5.3)
- **Step 4:** Task decomposition–identify tasks and subtasks (Tool: section 11.3.6; Example: section 11.5.4)
- **Step 5:** Assign workload ratings (Tool: section 11.3.7; Example: section 11.5.5)
- **Step 6:** Augment the task analysis with additional information (see section 11.3.8; Example: section 11.5.6)

This working example uses a series of tables to show how the practitioner might document the outcomes of each step. Table 24 to Table 26 show how to document roadway characteristics, segments, and tasks. Table 27 to Table 30 demonstrate, for one segment (i.e., Segment 3: Entry and Negotiation) how to decompose tasks into subtasks and document the subtask's information processing element (e.g., perceptual, cognitive, and psychomotor). Table 31 to Table 34 show how to assign each subtask a workload rating. In the full application of Approach 3, the practitioner would then create additional tables to document the subtasks for all roadway segments of interest, but these are not included for brevity. Therefore, Figure 106 to Figure 108 skip ahead to demonstrate the categorization of tasks (i.e., forced-paced versus self-paced) and development of the detailed workload estimates for all segments, even though the derivation of workload

Table 23.   The documented route information after the quantify roadway feature demands step is complete includes the derived roadway feature metrics and the total workload ticks for each column.

	1. Approach	2. Curve Discovery	3. Entry and Negotiation	4. Exit
Travel distance (ft)	100	250	700	200
Speed limit (mph)	35	35	35	35
Lane width (ft)	**10**	**10**	11	11
Shoulder width (ft)	4	4	**3**	5
Driveway frequency (#; #/mi)	1; 52.8	**4; 84.5**	1; 7.5	0; 0
Regulatory signs (#)	0	1	**7**	2
Warning signs (#)	0	0	0	1
% horizontal curve	0	0	**100%**	0
% grade	2%	**2.8%**	2.3%	0%
Unsignalized intersections	0	0	0	1
Bus stops	0	**1**	0	0
Total Workload Ticks	**1**	**4**	**3**	**2**

ratings for subtasks in Segments 1, 2, and 4 are not shown. The final presentation on workload relative to road segments is depicted in Figure 109.

Although this example focuses on a specific modality for succinctness, in practice, the practitioner might complete these steps to create multiple workload rating graphs that would cover the variety of modalities and road user populations relevant to the roadway under consideration.

11.5.1 Step 1. Collect Roadway Section Data

The roadway is characterized and documented using route maps, photographs, and videos collected by the practitioner (Figure 105). Static elements of interest (e.g., curve entry, signs) are identified, and their locations are documented (Table 24).

11.5.2 Step 2. Collect Analytical Data

Existing literature and reports that describe task analyses relevant to traversing a curve (Campbell et al., 2012) and heavy truck operation [Turanski and Tijerina, 1996; Washington State Department of Licensing (WDL), 2022] are identified. In this case, the practitioner did not have access to a heavy truck or truck drivers, so they did not record any driver-facing video of the facility.

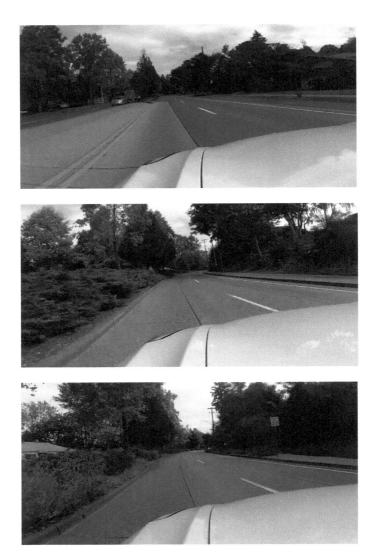

Figure 105.   Image stills from video captured by a GoPro camera affixed to the hood of the practitioner's vehicle (photos by Liberty Hoekstra-Atwood, 2020; used with permission).

Table 24. **The documented route information after the roadway-section data collection step is complete includes a schematic of the roadway of interest.**

Roadway Schematic

Roadway Feature ①
Milestone

Median ①
Milestone 1 - Curve is Visible
Milestone 2 - Curve Entry
Speed Limit Sign (35 mph) ②
Milestone 3 - Curve Exit
100 ft

Segments				
Key Driving Tasks				
Visual Demands and Information Sources				
Effective Information Modes				
Vehicle-Control Demands				
Primary Speed Influences				

Note: A blank template of this table is available in Chapter 12.

11.5.3 Step 3. Task Decomposition–Identify Segments

The curve is broken down into four primary segments, with each segment generally representing a related set of driving actions (Table 25).

11.5.4 Step 4. Task Decomposition–Identify Tasks and Subtasks

Driving tasks are then selected and decomposed successively into smaller activities to characterize how a heavy truck driver may traverse the curve (Table 26). Although not all tasks or subtasks identified in the task decomposition will be performed exhaustively by all heavy truck drivers, this list indicates reasonable tasks drivers are likely to perform to successfully navigate a section of roadway. Note that task decomposition is iterative. A practitioner may find value in reorganizing segments, tasks, or subtasks once they have produced an initial list. For brevity, the breakdown of tasks into subtasks is only shown for Segment 3: Entry and Negotiation (Table 27 to Table 30).

11.5.5 Step 5. Assign Workload Ratings

As shown in Table 20, within each task, workload values for subtasks are assigned based on a workload estimation tool for perceptual, cognitive, and psychomotor information processing demands in driving described in a previous FHWA report (Richard et al., 2006). As a first step,

Table 25.   The documented route information after the identify segments step is complete includes driving issues by roadway segment: visual demands, information modes, vehicle control, and speed issues.

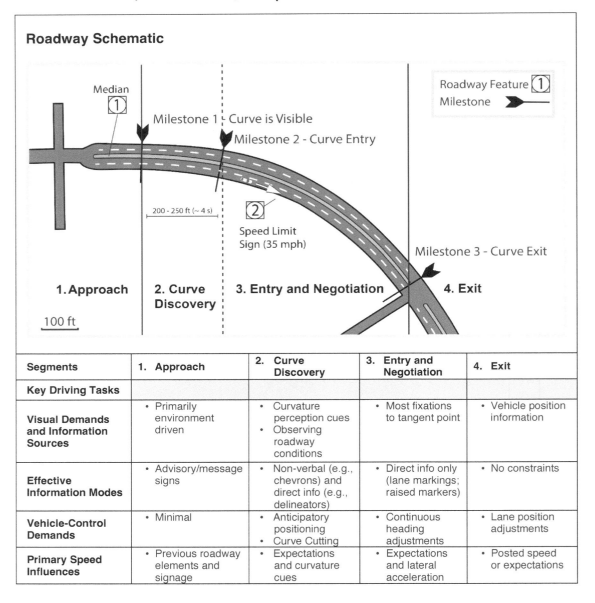

Segments	1. Approach	2. Curve Discovery	3. Entry and Negotiation	4. Exit
Key Driving Tasks				
Visual Demands and Information Sources	• Primarily environment driven	• Curvature perception cues • Observing roadway conditions	• Most fixations to tangent point	• Vehicle position information
Effective Information Modes	• Advisory/message signs	• Non-verbal (e.g., chevrons) and direct info (e.g., delineators)	• Direct info only (lane markings; raised markers)	• No constraints
Vehicle-Control Demands	• Minimal	• Anticipatory positioning • Curve Cutting	• Continuous heading adjustments	• Lane position adjustments
Primary Speed Influences	• Previous roadway elements and signage	• Expectations and curvature cues	• Expectations and lateral acceleration	• Posted speed or expectations

Table 26. After creating the road user task list, the documented route information is updated to include the key driving tasks that occur in each segment.

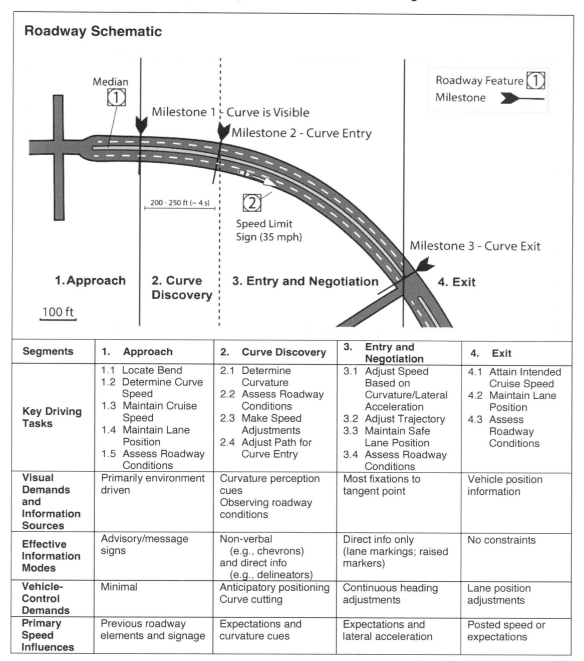

Segments	1. Approach	2. Curve Discovery	3. Entry and Negotiation	4. Exit
Key Driving Tasks	1.1 Locate Bend 1.2 Determine Curve Speed 1.3 Maintain Cruise Speed 1.4 Maintain Lane Position 1.5 Assess Roadway Conditions	2.1 Determine Curvature 2.2 Assess Roadway Conditions 2.3 Make Speed Adjustments 2.4 Adjust Path for Curve Entry	3.1 Adjust Speed Based on Curvature/Lateral Acceleration 3.2 Adjust Trajectory 3.3 Maintain Safe Lane Position 3.4 Assess Roadway Conditions	4.1 Attain Intended Cruise Speed 4.2 Maintain Lane Position 4.3 Assess Roadway Conditions
Visual Demands and Information Sources	Primarily environment driven	Curvature perception cues Observing roadway conditions	Most fixations to tangent point	Vehicle position information
Effective Information Modes	Advisory/message signs	Non-verbal (e.g., chevrons) and direct info (e.g., delineators)	Direct info only (lane markings; raised markers)	No constraints
Vehicle-Control Demands	Minimal	Anticipatory positioning Curve cutting	Continuous heading adjustments	Lane position adjustments
Primary Speed Influences	Previous roadway elements and signage	Expectations and curvature cues	Expectations and lateral acceleration	Posted speed or expectations

Table 27. Subtask breakdown for Segment 3, Task 3.1–Adjust speed based on curvature/lateral acceleration.

Task: Adjust Speed Based on Curvature/Lateral Acceleration (Campbell et al., 2012)	Workload Estimate	Process	Supplementary Notes
Subtask: Perceive curvature cues–lateral acceleration		Perceptual	Within the curve, the operator primarily uses heavy truck handling and lateral acceleration cues to adjust speed (Campbell et al., 2012).
Subtask: Determine speed adjustment		Cognitive	No supplementary notes.
Subtask: Accelerate slightly in the curve–foot on throttle or release throttle		Psychomotor	Accelerating in the curve helps the operator maintain control (WDL, 2022). Hard braking in a curve could be dangerous; the wheels can lock and cause a skid (WDL, 2022).

Note: A blank template of this table is available in Chapter 12.

Table 28. Subtask breakdown for Segment 3, Task 3.2–Adjust trajectory.

Task: Adjust Trajectory (Campbell et al., 2012)	Workload Estimate	Process	Supplementary Notes
Subtask: Perceive curvature cues–tangent point		Perceptual	During curve negotiation, the operator spends most of their visual resources looking at the tangent point, or the forward horizon on gradual curves, to keep the heavy truck aligned with the roadway (Campbell et al., 2012). Visual demands are highest in this segment and peak immediately after the point of curvature (Campbell et al., 2012). Therefore, communicating curve information in this segment could be done at the curve (e.g., lane markings) or within an area that operators could perceive with their peripheral vision (e.g., raised reflective markings in dark conditions) (Campbell et al., 2012).
Subtask: Determine target trajectory		Cognitive	No supplementary notes.
Subtask: Hold the steering wheel firmly with both hands		Psychomotor	The operator controls direction via the steering wheel (Turanski and Tijerina, 1996). If the heavy truck hits a curb or pothole, the operator can maintain a firm hold to continue steering (WDL, 2022).

Table 29. Subtask breakdown for Segment 3, Task 3.3–Maintain safe lane position.

Task: Maintain Lane Position (Richard et al., 2006)	Workload Estimate	Process	Supplementary Notes
Subtask: Visually observe the roadway ahead		Perceptual	The heavy truck operator can look at lane markings and road geometry and be aware of changes in the road scene (Turanski and Tijerina, 1996).
Subtask: Verify the correct lane position		Cognitive	No supplementary notes.
Subtask: Hold the steering wheel steady or adjust the steering		Psychomotor	The heavy truck operator controls direction, lane position, and spacing via the steering wheel (Turanski and Tijerina, 1996). They can make necessary adjustments to avoid over or under-steering the heavy truck (WDL, 2022). They may keep both hands on the steering wheel at all times unless they are actively shifting (WDL, 2022). In practice, heavy truck operators use only one hand for continuous steering 50% of the time (Kiger et al., 1992).

Table 30. Subtask breakdown for Segment 3, Task 3.4–Assess roadway conditions.

Task: Assess Roadway Conditions	Workload Estimate	Process	Supplementary Notes
Subtask: Look for potential hazards and obstacles ahead–visual; Listen for potential hazards–auditory		**Perceptual**	Heavy truck licensing materials advise that heavy truck operators look at least 12 to 15 seconds ahead (WDL, 2022). They can check upcoming traffic (WDL, 2022), lane markings, and road geometry, and be aware of changes in the road scene (the primary visual task) (Turanski and Tijerina, 1996). Changes in the road scene include monitoring weather, monitoring road conditions, and scanning for upcoming obstructions that may have been hidden on a roadway with a short sight distance (e.g., a curve or a hill).
Subtask: Monitor heavy truck cab for indications of potentially challenging driving conditions		**Perceptual**	Heavy truck licensing materials advise operators to follow up on cues (tactile, olfactory, visual, auditory) that indicate an issue with the heavy truck (WDL, 2022). Operators may glance at the gauges (Turanski and Tijerina, 1996) or the instrument panel to perceive these cues (e.g., a change in ambient weather conditions could be perceived by temperature information on the instrument panel, a thermometer, over the radio, or be physically perceived by the operator).
Subtask: Determine if perceptual cues indicate a potential crash or potentially challenging driving conditions		**Cognitive**	No supplementary notes.
Subtask: Turn head to glance at mirrors (Turanski and Tijerina, 1996)		**Psychomotor**	The operator turns their head to glance at either west coast (side) mirror (Turanski and Tijerina, 1996). The operator checks traffic in all directions (WDL, 2022). Quick mirror checks allow for visual attention to mainly focus on the road ahead (WDL, 2022).

the qualities of the subtask are matched to the description and examples in the reference table (Table 20) then the associated workload value is assigned (Table 31 to Table 34 outline how this would be done for the four tasks within Segment 3: Curve Entry and Negotiation). Workload values may be incremented if the subtask context is particularly complex [e.g., perceiving degraded signs or markings (Richard et al., 2006)].

11.5.6 Step 6. Augment the Task Analysis with Additional Information

To create workload estimation profiles (Figure 108), scenario segments were divided into four time intervals to help represent when a driver may perform a task within a segment (Figure 106). Tasks were then arranged into intervals based on their logical order or whether a driver could potentially perform the tasks concurrently. Tasks were also categorized based on whether they were forced-paced or self-paced. Next, the workload estimates from all tasks within each interval were summed. For example, to sum the workload estimates for Segment 3, Task 3.4—Assess roadway conditions, the practitioner would reference Table 24. Within this task, the ratings of the two perceptual subtasks sum to eight. This task has one cognitive subtask and one psychomotor subtask, so the summed cognitive workload and psychomotor workload ratings are 4 and 1 respectively.

Although self-paced tasks can be performed within any time interval within the driving segment, when tasks were self-paced rather than forced-paced, the workload for the task was only summed into the initial segment time interval where the driver could complete it (Figure 107). The summed workload ratings for concurrent perceptual, cognitive, and psychomotor tasks

Table 31. Subtask workload ratings for Segment 3, Task 3.1–Adjust speed based on curvature/lateral acceleration.

Task: Adjust Speed Based on Curvature/Lateral Acceleration	Workload Estimate	Process	Supplementary Notes
Subtask: Perceive curvature cues–lateral acceleration	1	**Perceptual** This subtask involves registering motion.	Within the curve, the operator primarily uses heavy truck handling and lateral acceleration cues to adjust speed.
Subtask: Determine speed adjustment	4	**Cognitive** This subtask involves the evaluation of and judgment about a single aspect.	No supplementary notes.
Subtask: Accelerate slightly in the curve–foot on throttle or release throttle	3	**Psychomotor** This subtask involves a continuous adjustment action.	Accelerating inside the curve can help the operator maintain control. Braking in a curve is dangerous; the wheels can lock and cause a skid.

Table 32. Subtask workload ratings for Segment 3, Task 3.2–Adjust trajectory.

Task: Adjust Trajectory	Workload Estimate	Process	Supplementary Notes
Subtask: Perceive curvature cues–tangent point	5	**Perceptual** This subtask involves visually tracking curvature cues.	During curve negotiation, the operator spends most of their visual resources looking at the tangent point, or the forward horizon, on gradual curves to keep the heavy truck aligned with the roadway. Visual demands are highest in this segment and peak immediately after the point of curvature. Therefore, communicating curve information in this segment could be done at the curve (e.g., lane markings) or within an area that operators could perceive with their peripheral vision (e.g., raised reflective markings in dark conditions).
Subtask: Determine target trajectory	4	**Cognitive** This subtask involves the evaluation of and judgment about a single aspect.	No supplementary notes.
Subtask: Hold the steering wheel firmly with both hands	3	**Psychomotor** This subtask involves a continuous adjustment action.	The operator controls direction via the steering wheel. If the heavy truck hits a curb or pothole, the operator can maintain a firm hold to continue steering.

Table 33.   Subtask workload ratings for Segment 3, Task 3.3–Maintain safe lane position.

Task: Maintain Lane Position	Workload Estimate	Process	Supplementary Notes
Subtask: Visually observe the roadway ahead	1	**Perceptual** This subtask involves registering vehicle heading.	The heavy truck operator can look at lane markings and road geometry and be aware of changes in the road scene.
Subtask: Verify the correct lane position	1	**Cognitive** This subtask involves a simple conditioned response.	No supplementary notes.
Subtask: Hold the steering wheel steady or adjust the steering	3	**Psychomotor** This subtask involves a continuous adjustment action.	The heavy truck operator controls direction, lane position, and spacing via the steering wheel. They can make necessary adjustments to avoid over or under-steering the heavy truck, and they may keep both hands on the steering wheel at all times unless they are actively shifting. In practice, heavy truck operators use only one hand for continuous steering 50% of the time.

Table 34.   Subtask workload ratings for Segment 3, Task 3.4–Assess roadway conditions.

Task: Assess Roadway Conditions	Workload Estimate	Process	Supplementary Notes
Subtask: Look for potential hazards and obstacles ahead–visual; Listen for potential hazards–auditory	7	**Perceptual** This subtask involves scanning for potential obstacles and hazards and listening for unsafe situations.	Heavy truck licensing materials advise that heavy truck operators look at least 12 to 15 seconds ahead. They can check upcoming traffic, lane markings, and road geometry and be aware of changes in the road scene (the primary visual task). Changes in the road scene include monitoring weather, monitoring road conditions, and scanning for upcoming obstructions that may have been hidden on a roadway with a short sight distance (e.g., a curve or a hill).
Subtask: Monitor heavy truck cab for indications of potentially challenging driving conditions	1	**Perceptual** This subtask involves detecting visual, auditory, or olfactory stimuli.	Heavy truck licensing materials advise operators to follow up on cues (tactile, olfactory, visual, auditory) that indicate an issue with the heavy truck. Operators may glance at the gauges or the instrument panel to perceive these cues (e.g., a change in ambient weather conditions could be perceived by temperature information on the instrument panel, a thermometer, over the radio, or be physically perceived by the operator).
Subtask: Determine if perceptual cues indicate safe or unsafe conditions	4	**Cognitive** This subtask involves the evaluation of and judgment about a single aspect.	No supplementary notes.
Subtask: Turn head to glance at mirrors	1	**Psychomotor** This subtask involves a simple automatic behavior.	The operator turns their head to glance at either west coast (side) mirror. The operator checks traffic in all directions. Quick mirror checks allow for visual attention to mainly focus on the road ahead.

Segment	Task	Summed Workload Ratings for Perceptual Subtasks	Summed Workload Ratings for Cognitive Subtasks	Summed Workload Ratings for Psychomotor Subtasks	Time Interval 1	Time Interval 2	Time Interval 3	Time Interval 4
1. Curve Approach	1.1 Locate Bend	9	4	0	S	/-->	/-->	
	1.2 Determine Curve Speed	10	7	0		S	/-->	/-->
	1.3 Maintain Cruise Speed	3	4	3	F			
	1.4 Maintain Lane Position	1	1	3	F			
	1.5 Assess Roadway Conditions	8	4	1	F			
2. Curve Discovery	2.1 Determine Curvature	8	6	0	F			
	2.2 Assess Roadway Conditions	8	4	1				
	2.3 Make Speed Adjustments	0	6	3		F		
	2.4 Adjust Path for Curve Entry	0	4	3				F
3. Curve Entry & Negotiation	3.1 Adjust Speed Based on Curvature/Lateral Acceleration	1	4	3	F			
	3.2 Adjust Trajectory	5	4	3		F		
	3.3 Maintain Lane Position	1	1	3	F			
	3.4 Assess Roadway Conditions	8	4	1	F			
4. Curve Exit	4.1 Attain Desired Cruise Speed	3	4	3	S	/-->	/-->	
	4.2 Maintain Lane Position	1	1	3	F			
	4.3 Assess Roadway Conditions	8	4	1	F			
					F = Force-paced tasks			
					S = Self-paced tasks			

Note: A blank template of this figure is available in Chapter 12.

Figure 106.   Subtask workload ratings are summed for each task. The tasks are categorized as forced-paced tasks or self-paced tasks and are then arranged into time intervals based on their logical sequence and pacing.

	1. Curve Approach			
	9 /-->	/-->		
		10 /-->	/-->	
	3	3	3	3
	1	1	1	1
	8	8	8	8
Total relative perceptual workload for Segment 1	21	22	12	12

Note: A blank template of this figure is available in Chapter 12.

Figure 107.   An example of how relative workload is derived for each segment based on task arrangements. When tasks were self-paced rather than forced-paced, the workload for the task was only summed into the initial segment time interval where the driver could complete it.

(Figure 108) were used to create a workload profile for the entire roadway of interest (Figure 109). Peaks in the workload profile in the unshaded regions indicate where multiple demands incurred by the driver from the roadway environment may peak and create information processing bottlenecks reflecting high workload/demands. The implication of these workload rating peaks is that adding additional load (e.g., complex signage) in these peak areas, especially of the same demand type (e.g., perceptual) is more likely to lead to scenarios where drivers do not have the resources to process the roadway. Peaks in the workload profile in the gray-shaded regions indicate where information bottlenecks could occur because of driving task demands, but because of one or more of the driving tasks being self-paced, drivers may be able to allocate resources optimally in these regions to avoid overload.

The purpose of this method is not to draw firm conclusions about driver performance or vehicle safety from the workload values but rather to identify intervals within each scenario where the workload is higher relative to other intervals. The derived workload profile can help a designer identify parts of the roadway where multiple factors (e.g., forced-paced tasks and high workload) may converge to create potential information processing bottlenecks (Richard et al., 2006).

In this example, demands on a heavy truck driver's perceptual processes are relatively high and temporally constrained at the beginning of the Curve Discovery and throughout the Curve Entry and Negotiation tasks. A practical application of this information would be to avoid putting complex signage in locations where these tasks occur to increase the likelihood that drivers will perceive the signs and reduce the likelihood of task interference. Note that if the practitioners augmented this work with direct observation (e.g., video, eye tracking) to observe real drivers traversing the roadway, it would be possible to identify instances of overload and underload through those observations or through changes in driving performance (e.g., Gawron, 2000; Matthews and Reinerman-Jones, 2017).

Segment	Time interval	Summed Workload Ratings for Concurrent Perceptual Tasks	Summed Workload Ratings for Concurrent Cognitive Tasks	Summed Workload Ratings for Concurrent Psychomotor Tasks	Summed Workload Ratings for All Concurrent Tasks
1. Curve Approach	1	21	13	7	41
	2	22	16	7	45
	3	12	9	7	28
	4	12	9	7	28
2. Curve Discovery	1	16	10	1	27
	2	8	10	4	22
	3	8	10	4	22
	4	8	8	4	20
3. Curve Entry & Negotiation	1	10	9	7	26
	2	15	13	10	38
	3	14	9	7	30
	4	14	9	7	30
4. Curve Exit	1	12	9	7	28
	2	9	5	4	18
	3	9	5	4	18
	4	9	5	4	18

Note: A blank template of this figure is available in Chapter 12.

Figure 108. Workload ratings are summed by intervals for perceptual, cognitive, and psychomotor demands.

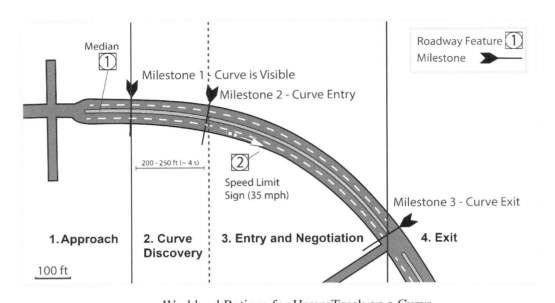

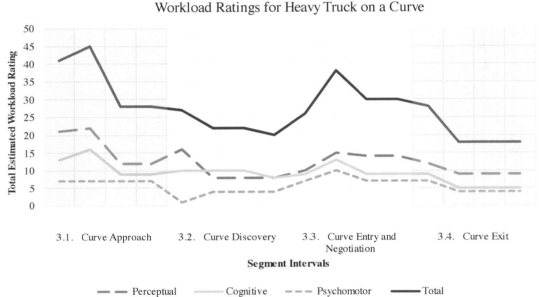

Figure 109. *Workload profile for the heavy truck on a curve scenario. The intervals containing only forced-paced tasks are shaded in white, while intervals that contain at least one self-paced task are shaded in gray. Peaks in the workload profile in the gray-shaded regions indicate where information bottlenecks could occur because of driving task demands, but because of one or more of the driving tasks being self-paced, drivers may be able to allocate resources optimally in these regions to avoid overload.*

CHAPTER 12

Blank Templates and Worksheets

This chapter contains blank template versions (Table 35 to Table 40) of tables and figures shown in other chapters. Practitioners can use these tables to perform the diagnostic procedures described in this toolset.

Table 35. A blank template for the Haddon Matrix as shown in Chapter 3, Table 5.

Phases	Factors					
	Human	Vehicle	Physical Environment/ Context	Social Environment	User-Mix Considerations	Interactions Between Users
Pre-event *(Before the crash occurs)* **Factors that may increase the likelihood of the crash before the crash event**	•	•	•	•	•	•
Event *(During the crash)* **Factors that may influence the injury or severity of the crash during the crash event**	•	•	•	•	•	•
Post-event *(After the crash)* **Factors that may influence the survivability of the crash after the event**	•	•	•	•	•	•

Note: This blank template is suitable for identifying factors related to personal attributes, vehicle attributes, and environmental attributes before, during, and after an injury or death to help generate ideas on crash prevention and countermeasure implementation.

Table 36.   A blank template from Table 24 in Chapter 11.

Roadway Schematic				
Segments				
Key Driving Tasks				
Visual Demands and Information Sources				
Effective Information Modes				
Vehicle-Control Demands				
Primary Speed Influences				

Note: This template is suitable for documenting route information during the Collect Roadway Section Data process (section 11.3.1 in Chapter 11) and the Task Decomposition—Identify Segments process (section 11.3.5 in Chapter 11).

Table 37.   A blank template version of Table 27 in Chapter 11.

Task:	Workload Estimate (e.g., Table 20)	Process (Perceptual, Cognitive, Psychomotor)	Supplementary Notes
Subtask:			
Subtask:			
Subtask:			
Subtask:			

Note: During the Task Decomposition—Identify Tasks and Subtasks process (section 11.3.6 in Chapter 11), this template is suitable for identifying tasks and subtasks.

Table 38.   A blank template version of Figure 106 in Chapter 11.

Segment	Task	Summed Workload Ratings for Perceptual Subtasks	Summed Workload Ratings for Cognitive Subtasks	Summed Workload Ratings for Psychomotor Subtasks	Time Interval 1	Time Interval 2	Time Interval 3	Time Interval 4
1.	1.1							
	1.2							
	1.3							
	1.4							
	1.5							

Note: This template is suitable for calculating summed workload ratings across workload type during the Assign Workload Values process (section 11.3.7 in Chapter 11) and for documenting forced- and self-paced tasks within segment time intervals during the Augment the Task Analysis with Additional Information process (section 11.3.8 in Chapter 11).

Table 39.   A blank template version of Figure 107 in Chapter 11.

1. *Segment Name*	Interval 1	Interval 2	Interval 3	Interval 4
Total relative perceptual workload for Segment 1				

Note: During the Assign Workload Values process (section 11.3.7 in Chapter 11), this template is suitable for calculating summed workload ratings within segment time intervals.

Table 40.   A blank template version of Figure 108 in Chapter 11.

Segment	Time interval	Summed Workload Ratings for Concurrent Perceptual Tasks	Summed Workload Ratings for Concurrent Cognitive Tasks	Summed Workload Ratings for Concurrent Psychomotor Tasks	Summed Workload Ratings for All Concurrent Tasks
1.	1				
	2				
	3				
	4				

Note: During the Assign Workload Values process (section 11.3.7 in Chapter 11), this template is suitable for documenting the summed workload ratings for each workload type within each segment time interval.

References

Able, S., J. Lindley, and J. Paniati. (2021). Safe System Strategic Plan (No. FHWA-SA-21-088). U.S. Department of Transportation, Federal Highway Administration, Washington, DC.

Albee, M., and F. Gross. (2021). HSIP 2019 National Summary Report (No. FHWA-SA-21-006). U.S. Department of Transportation, Federal Highway Administration, Washington, DC.

Albin, R., V. Brinkly, J. Cheung, F. Julian, C. Satterfield, W. Stein, E. Donnell, H. McGee, A. Holzem, M. Albee, J. Wood, and F. Hanscom. (2016). Low-Cost Treatments for Horizontal Curve Safety 2016 (No. FHWA-SA-15-084). U.S. Department of Transportation, Federal Highway Administration, Washington, DC.

Alexander, G. J., and H. Lunenfeld. (1986). Driver Expectancy in Highway Design and Operations (No. FHWA-TO-86-1). U.S. Department of Transportation, Federal Highway Administration, Washington, DC.

American Association of State Highway and Transportation Officials (AASHTO). (2010). *Highway Safety Manual*. American Association of State Highway and Transportation Officials, Washington, DC. https://www.highwaysafetymanual.org/Pages/default.aspx.

American Association of State Highway and Transportation Officials (AASHTO). (2018). A Policy on Geometric Design of Highways and Streets. American Association of State Highway and Transportation Officials, Washington, DC.

American Association of State Highway and Transportation Officials (AASHTO). (n.d.a). SHRP2 Safety Solutions. American Association of State Highway and Transportation Officials, Washington, DC. https://shrp2.transportation.org/Pages/Safety.aspx.

American Association of State Highway and Transportation Officials (AASHTO). (n.d.b). Transportation Systems Management and Operations Guidance. American Association of State Highway and Transportation Officials, Washington, DC.

Angell, L., J. Auflick, P. A. Austria, D. Kochhar, L. Tijerina, W. Biever, T. Diptiman, J. Hogsett, and S. Kiger. (2006). Driver Workload Metrics Project. Final Report. DOT HS 810 635. U.S. Department of Transportation, National Highway Traffic Safety Administration, Washington, DC.

Antonucci, N. D., K. K. Hardy, J. E. Bryden, T. R. Neuman, R. Pfefer, and K. Slack. (2005). *NCHRP Report 500, Volume 17: A Guide for Reducing Work Zone Collisions*. Transportation Research Board of the National Academies, Washington, DC.

American Road and Transportation Builders Association (ARTBA). (2024). National Work Zone Safety Information Clearinghouse, Texas A&M Transportation Institute, College Station, TX. https://workzonesafety.org.

Blackburn, L., C. Zegeer, and K. Brookshire. (2018). Field Guide for Selecting Countermeasures at Uncontrolled Pedestrian Crossing Locations (No. FHWA-SA-18-018). U.S. Department of Transportation, Federal Highway Administration, Washington, DC.

Brewer, M., and L. Bedsole. (2015). Desk Reference to the Handbook for Designing Roadways for the Aging Population (No. FHWA-SA-15-088). U.S. Department of Transportation, Federal Highway Administration, Washington, DC.

Brown, J. L., D. M. Prendez, J. Lee, A. Romo, J. L. Campbell, J. Hutton, I. Potts, and D. Torbic. (2021). *NCHRP Web-Only Document 316: Human Factors Guidelines for Road Systems 2021 Update, Volume 1: Updated and New Chapters*. Transportation Research Board, Washington, DC. https://doi.org/10.17226/26473.

Campbell, J. L., J. B. Richman, C. Carney, and J. D. Lee. (2004). *In-Vehicle Display Icons and Other Information Elements, Volume I: Guidelines* (FHWA-RD-03-065). U.S. Department of Transportation, Federal Highway Administration, Washington, DC. https://www.fhwa.dot.gov/publications/research/safety/03065/03065.pdf.

Campbell, J. L., M. G. Lichty, J. L. Brown, C. M. Richard, J. Graving, J. Graham, M. O'Laughlin, and D. Harwood. (2012). *NCHRP Report 600: Human Factors Guidelines for Road Systems, Second Edition*. Transportation Research Board of the National Academies, Washington, DC. https://www.trb.org/Main/Blurbs/167909.aspx.

Campbell, J. L., R. Hull, and A. Maistros. (2018). Primer on the Joint Use of the Highway Safety Manual (HSM) and the Human Factors Guidelines (HFG) for Road Systems. NCHRP Project 20-07 [334]. Battelle, Columbus, OH. https://onlinepubs.trb.org/Onlinepubs/NCHRP/docs/NCHRP20-07_334Primer.pdf.

Charman, S., G. Grayson, S. Helman, J. Kennedy, O. de Smidt, B. Lawton, G. Nossek, L. Wiesauer, A. Furdos, V. Pelikan, P. Skladany, P. Pokorny, M. Matějka, and P. Tučka. (2010). Self-Explaining Roads: Literature Review and Treatment Information. SPACE project Deliverable 1.

Choi, E. H. (2010). Crash Factors in Intersection-Related Crashes: An On-Scene Perspective. (No. DOT HS-811 366). U.S. Department of Transportation, National Highway Traffic Safety Administration, Washington, DC.

Coury, B. G., V. S. Ellingstad, and J. M. Kolly. (2010). Transportation Accident Investigation: The Development of Human Factors Research and Practice. Reviews of Human Factors and Ergonomics, Vol. 6, No. 11: 1–33.

Dewar, R., and P. Olson. (2007). Human Factors in Traffic Safety (2nd ed.). Lawyers and Judges Publishing Company, Inc., Tucson, AZ.

Dingus, T. A., S. G. Klauer, V. L. Neale, A. Petersen, S. E. Lee, J. Sudweeks, M. A. Perez, J. Hankey, D. Ramsey, S. Gupta, C. Butcher, Z. R. Doerzaph, J. Jermeland, and R. R. Knipling. (2006). The 100-Car Naturalistic Driving Study, Phase II-Results of the 100-Car Field Experiment (No. DOT-HS-810-593). U.S. Department of Transportation, National Highway Traffic Safety Administration, Washington, DC.

Dong, Y., and J. S. Wood. (2023). Evaluation of Crash Contributing Factors. engrXiv [Preprint]. https://doi.org/10.31224/2942.

Dunn, N. J., J. S. Hickman, and R. J. Hanowski. (2014). Crash Trifecta: A Complex Driving Scenario Describing Crash Causation. Advances in Human Aspects of Transportation, Vol. 3, No. 9: 369.

Edquist, J., and I. Johnston. (2008). Visual Clutter in Road Environments—What it Does, and What to do About It. 2008 Australasian Road Safety Research Policing and Education Conference, Adelaide, South Australia.

Falkmer, T., and N. P. Gregersen. (2005). A Comparison of Eye Movement Behavior of Inexperienced and Experienced Drivers in Real Traffic Environments. Optometry and Vision Science, Vol. 82, No. 8: 732–739.

Fambro, D. B., R. J. Koppa, D. L. Picha, and K. Fitzpatrick. (1998). Driver Perception-Brake Response in Stopping Sight Distance Situations. Transportation Research Record: Journal of the Transportation Research Board, No. 1628: 1–7.

Federal Highway Administration (FHWA). (2009). Manual on Uniform Traffic Control Devices (MUTCD). U.S. Department of Transportation, Federal Highway Administration, Washington, DC.

Federal Highway Administration (FHWA). (2010). FHWA Highway Safety Improvement Program Manual. U.S. Department of Transportation, Federal Highway Administration, Washington, DC.

Federal Highway Administration (FHWA). (2016). Strategic Highway Safety Plan (SHSP) Guidance. U.S. Department of Transportation, Federal Highway Administration, Office of Safety, Washington, DC.

Federal Highway Administration (FHWA). (2022a). Nighttime Visibility. U.S. Department of Transportation, Federal Highway Administration, Washington, DC. https://highways.dot.gov/safety/other/visibility/nighttime-visibility.

Federal Highway Administration (FHWA). (2022b). Vulnerable Road User Safety Assessment. U.S. Department of Transportation, Federal Highway Administration, Washington, DC. https://highways.dot.gov/sites/fhwa.dot.gov/files/2022-10/VRU%20Safety%20Assessment%20Guidance%20FINAL_508.pdf.

Federal Highway Administration (FHWA). (2022c). Corridor Access Management (U.S. DOT Report No. FHWA-SA-21-040). U.S. Department of Transportation, Federal Highway Administration, Washington, DC. https://highways.dot.gov/sites/fhwa.dot.gov/files/2022-06/12_Corridor%20Access%20Management_508.pdf.

Federal Highway Administration (FHWA). (2023a). HSIP State Reports: 2021. U.S. Department of Transportation, Federal Highway Administration, Washington, DC. https://highways.dot.gov/safety/hsip/hsip-state-reports-2021.

Federal Highway Administration (FHWA). (2023b). Interactive Highway Safety Design Model (IHSDM): Overview. U.S. Department of Transportation, Federal Highway Administration, Washington, DC. https://highways.dot.gov/research/safety/interactive-highway-safety-design-model/interactive-highway-safety-design-model-ihsdm-overview.

Federal Highway Administration (FHWA). (2023c). Pedestrian and Bicycle Crash Analysis Tool (PBCAT). Highway Safety Information System (HSIS). U.S. Department of Transportation, Federal Highway Administration, Washington, DC. https://highways.dot.gov/research/pbcat/overview.

Federal Highway Administration (FHWA). (2024). Welcome to Road Weather Management. U.S. Department of Transportation, Federal Highway Administration, Washington, DC. https://ops.fhwa.dot.gov/weather/.

Federal Highway Administration (FHWA). (n.d.a). Bicycle Safety Guide and Countermeasure Selection System (BIKESAFE). U.S. Department of Transportation, Federal Highway Administration, Washington, DC. http://www.pedbikesafe.org/bikesafe/

Federal Highway Administration (FHWA). (n.d.b). Developing CMFs. Crash Modification Factors Clearinghouse. U.S. Department of Transportation, Federal Highway Administration, Washington, DC. www.cmfclearinghouse.org/developing_cmfs.cfm.

Federal Highway Administration (FHWA). (n.d.c). Pedestrian Safety Guide and Countermeasure Selection System (PEDSAFE). U.S. Department of Transportation, Federal Highway Administration, Washington, DC. http://www.pedbikesafe.org/PEDSAFE/.

Federal Highway Administration (FHWA). (n.d.d). Proven Safety Countermeasures. U.S. Department of Transportation, Federal Highway Administration, Washington, DC. https://highways.dot.gov/safety/proven-safety-countermeasures.

Finkel, E., C. McCormick, M. Mitman, S. Abel, and J. Clark. (2020). Integrating the Safe System Approach with the Highway Safety Improvement Program: An Informational Report (No. FHWA-SA-20-018). U.S. Department of Transportation, Federal Highway Administration, Office of Safety, Washington, DC.

Fitzpatrick, K., M. D. Wooldridge, O. Tsimhoni, J. M. Collins, P. Green, K. M. Bauer, I. B. Anderson, L. Elefteriadou, D. W. Harwood, N. Irizarry, R. Koppa, R. A. Krammes, J. McFadden, K. D. Parma, K. Passetti and B. Poggioli. (2000). Alternative Design Consistency Rating Methods for Two-Lane Rural Highways (No. FHWA-RD-99-172). U.S. Department of Transportation, Federal Highway Administration, Washington, DC.

Francis, E. L., R. A. Tyrrell, and D. A. Owens. (2020). Perception Response Time and Its Misapplication: An Historical and Forensic Perspective. *Theoretical Issues in Ergonomics Science* Vol. 21, No. 3: 327–346.

Garber, N. J., and M. Zhao. (2002). Crash Characteristics at Work Zones (VTRC 02-R12). Virginia Transportation Research Council, Charlottesville, VA.

Gartner, W. B., and M. R. Murphy. (1979). Concepts of Workload. In: B. O. Hartman and R. E. McKenzie (Eds.), *Survey of Methods to Assess Workload*. Advisory Group for Aerospace Research and Development (AGARD), USAF School of Aerospace Medicine, Brooks Air Force Base, TX.

Gawron, V. J. (2000). *Human Performance Measures Handbook*. Lawrence Erlbaum Associates Publishers, Mahwah, NJ.

Gross, F. (2017). Highway Safety Improvement Program (HSIP) Evaluation Guide. FHWA-SA-17-039. U.S. Department of Transportation, Federal Highway Administration, Office of Safety, Washington, DC. https://highways.dot.gov/sites/fhwa.dot.gov/files/2022-06/fhwasa17039.pdf.

Habib, K., A. Shalkamy, and K. El-Basyouny. (2019). Investigating the Effects of Mental Workload on Highway Safety. *Transportation Research Record: Journal of the Transportation Research Board,* No. 2673: 619–629.

Haddon, W. (1972). A Logical Framework for Categorizing Highway Safety Phenomena and Activity. *Journal of Trauma*, Vol. 12: 193–207.

Haddon, W. (1980). Advances in the Epidemiology of Injuries as a Basis for Public Policy. *Public Health Reports*, Vol. 95: 411–421.

Hamilton, D. B., C. R. Bierbaum, and L. A. Fulford. (1991). Task Analysis/Workload (TAWL). User's Guide: Version 4.0 (Research Product 91-11). Anacapa Sciences, Inc., U.S. Army Research Institute, Aviation R&D Activity, U.S. Army Research Institute for the Behavioral and Social Sciences, Fort Rucker, AL.

Harwood, D. W., D. J. Torbic, K. R. Richard, and M. M. Meyer. (2010). Safety Analyst TM: Software Tools for Safety Management of Specific Highway Sites. FHWA-HRT-10-063. U.S. Department of Transportation, Federal Highway Administration, Washington, DC.

Hauer, E. (1997). *Observational Before-After Studies in Road Safety: Estimating the Effect of Highway and Traffic Engineering Measures on Road Safety*. Emerald Group Publishing, Bingley, UK.

Hauer, E. (2020). Crash Causation and Prevention. *Accident Analysis and Prevention,* Vol. 143: 105528.

Hills, B. L. (1980). Vision, Visibility, and Perception in Driving. *Perception*, Vol. 9: 183–216.

Kane, M. R., L. E. King, K. A. Buch, and M. L. Carpenter. (1999). Motorists' Perception of Work Zone Safety. FHWA/NC-99-006. North Carolina Department of Transportation, Charlotte, NC.

Kiger, S., T. Rockwell, S. Niswonger, L. Tijerna, L. Myers, and T. Nygren. (1992). Heavy Vehicle Driver Workload Assessment – Task 3: Task Analysis Data Collection. DOT HS 808 467 [3]. U.S. Department of Transportation, National Highway Traffic Safety Administration, Washington, DC.

Klauer, S. G., T. A. Dingus, V. L. Neale, J. D. Sudweeks, and D. J. Ramsey. (2006). The Impact of Driver Inattention on Near-Crash/Crash Risk: An Analysis Using the 100-Car Naturalistic Driving Study Data. DOT HS 810 594. U.S. Department of Transportation, National Highway Traffic Safety Administration, Washington, DC.

Krammes, R. A., and S. W. Glascock. (1992). Geometric Inconsistencies and Accident Experience on Two-Lane Rural Highways. *Transportation Research Record*, No. 1356.

Krauss, D. A. (2015). *Forensic Aspects of Driver Perception and Response*. Lawyers and Judges Publishing Company, Inc., Tucson, AZ.

Lerner, N. D., R. E. Llaneras, H. W. McGee, S. Taori, and F. Alexander. (2003). *NCHRP Report 488: Additional Investigations on Driver Information Overload*. Transportation Research Board of the National Academies, Washington, DC.

Li, Y., and Y. Bai. (2008). Comparison of Characteristics Between Fatal and Injury Accidents in the Highway Construction Zones. *Safety Science*, Vol. 46: 646–660.

Liu, C., and R. Subramanian. (2009). Factors Related to Fatal Single-Vehicle Run-Off-Road Crashes. DOT HS 811 232. National Center for Statistics and Analysis, Mathematical Analysis Division, U.S. Department of Transportation, National Highway Traffic Safety Administration, Washington, DC.

Liu, C., and T. J. Ye. (2011). Run-Off-Road Crashes: An On-Scene Perspective. HS 811 500. National Center for Statistics and Analysis, Mathematical Analysis Division, U.S. Department of Transportation, National Highway Traffic Safety Administration, Washington, DC.

Lunenfeld, H., and G. J. Alexander. (1990). A User's Guide to Positive Guidance. FHWA-SA-90-017. U.S. Department of Transportation, Federal Highway Administration, Washington, DC.

Martens, M., S. Comte, and N. Kaptein. (1997). The Effects of Road Design on Speed Behaviour: A Literature Review. TNO Report TM 97 B021. TNO Human Factors Research Institute, the Netherlands.

Matthews, G., and L. Reinerman-Jones. (2017). Workload Assessment: How to Diagnose Workload Issues and Enhance Performance. Human Factors and Ergonomics Society, Santa Monica, CA.

McLaughlin, S. B., J. M. Hankey, S. G. Klauer, and T. A. Dingus. (2009). Contributing Factors to Run-Off-Road Crashes and Near-Crashes. Report DOT HS 811 079. U.S. Department of Transportation, National Highway Traffic Safety Administration, Office of Human-Vehicle Performance Research, Washington, DC.

Messer, C. J. (1980). Methodology for Evaluating Geometric Design Consistency. *Transportation Research Record: Journal of the Transportation Research Board*, No. 757.

Messer, C. J., J. M. Mounce, and R. Q. Brackett. (1979). Highway Geometric Design Consistency Related to Driver Expectancy, Volume III, Methodology for Evaluating Geometric Design Consistency. Report No. FHWA/RD-81/037. U.S. Department of Transportation, Federal Highway Administration, Washington, DC.

Muttart, J. W. (2005). Estimating Driver Response Times. *Handbook of Human Factors in Litigation*. CRC Press, Boca Raton, FL.

National Association of City Transportation Officials (NACTO). (2013). *Urban Street Design Guide*. Island Press, Washington, DC.

National Association of City Transportation Officials (NACTO). (2014). *Urban Bikeway Design Guide*. Island Press, Washington, DC.

National Center for Statistics and Analysis (NCSA). (2023a). Pedestrians: 2021 Data. Traffic Safety Facts. Report No. DOT HS 813 458. U.S. Department of Transportation, National Highway Traffic Safety Administration, Washington, DC.

National Center for Statistics and Analysis (NCSA). (2023b). Bicyclists and Other Cyclists: 2021 Data. Traffic Safety Facts. Report No. DOT HS 813 484. U.S. Department of Transportation, National Highway Traffic Safety Administration, Washington, DC.

National Committee for Injury Prevention and Control. (1989). *Injury Prevention: Meeting the Challenge*. Oxford University Press, Oxford, United Kingdom.

National Highway Traffic Safety Administration (NHTSA). (2008a). National Motor Vehicle Crash Causation Survey. Report to Congress. No. DOT HS 811 059. U.S. Department of Transportation, National Highway Traffic Safety Administration, Washington, DC.

National Highway Traffic Safety Administration (NHTSA). (2008b). Traffic Safety Facts 2008. DOT HS 811 170. U.S. Department of Transportation, National Highway Traffic Safety Administration, Washington, DC.

National Highway Traffic Safety Administration (NHTSA). (n.d.a). Bicycle Safety. U.S. Department of Transportation, National Highway Traffic Safety Administration, Washington, DC. https://www.nhtsa.gov/road-safety/bicycle-safety.

National Highway Traffic Safety Administration (NHTSA). (n.d.b). Crash Investigation Sampling System: Motor Vehicle Crash Data Collection. U.S. Department of Transportation, National Highway Traffic Safety Administration, Washington, DC.

National Highway Traffic Safety Administration (NHTSA). (n.d.c). Fatality Analysis Reporting System (FARS). U.S. Department of Transportation, National Highway Traffic Safety Administration, Washington, DC. https://www.nhtsa.gov/research-data/fatality-analysis-reporting-system-fars.

National Highway Traffic Safety Administration (NHTSA). (n.d.d). National Automotive Sampling System. U.S. Department of Transportation, National Highway Traffic Safety Administration, Washington, DC.

National Transportation Safety Board (NTSB). (2004). Rear-End Collision and Subsequent Vehicle Intrusion into Pedestrian Space at Certified Farmer's Market. Highway Accident Report TSB/HAR-04/04, PB2004-916204. National Transportation Safety Board, Washington, DC.

National Transportation Safety Board (NTSB). (2009). Pedal Misapplication in Heavy Vehicles. Highway Special Investigation Report NTSB/SIR-09/02. National Transportation Safety Board, Washington, DC.

Olson, P. L., and M. Sivak. (1986). Perception-Response Time to Unexpected Roadway Hazards. *Human Factors* Vol. 28, No. 1: 91–96.

Olson, P. L., K. Campbell, D. Massie, D. S. Battle, E. C. Traube, T. Aoki, T. Sato, and L. C. Pettis. (1992). Performance Requirements for Large Truck Conspicuity Enhancements. Report No. UMTRI-92-8. University of Michigan, Ann Arbor, MI.

Permanent International Association of Road Congresses (PIARC). (2012). Human Factors in Road Design: Review of Design Standards in Nine Countries. World Road Association, Permanent International Association of Road Congresses, Paris, France.

Permanent International Association of Road Congresses (PIARC). (2016). Human Factors Guidelines for a Safer Man-Road Interface. World Road Association, Permanent International Association of Road Congresses, Paris, France.

Permanent International Association of Road Congresses (PIARC). (2019a). Road Safety Manual, a Guide for Practitioners: Planning, Design, and Evaluation. World Road Association, Permanent International Association of Road Congresses, Paris, France.

Permanent International Association of Road Congresses (PIARC). (2019b). Vulnerable Road Users: Diagnosis of Design and Operational Safety Problems and Potential Countermeasures. World Road Association, Permanent International Association of Road Congresses, Paris, France.

Pomerleau, D., T. Jochem, C. Thorpe, P. Batavia, D. Pape, J. Hadden, N. J. McMillan, N. Brown, and J. H. Everson. (1999). Run-Off-Road Collision Avoidance Using IVHS Countermeasures. DOT HS 809 170. U.S. Department of Transportation, National Highway Traffic Safety Administration, Washington, DC.

Preston, H., R. Storm, J. D. Bennett, and B. Wemple. (2013). Systemic Safety Project Selection Tool. FHWA-SA-13-019. U.S. Department of Transportation, Federal Highway Administration, Washington, DC.

Pullen-Seufert, N. C., and W. L. Hall. (2008). The Art of Appropriate Evaluation: A Guide for Highway Safety Program Managers. DOT HS 811 061. U.S. Department of Transportation, National Highway Traffic Safety Administration, Washington, DC.

Reason, J. (1995). Understanding Adverse Events: Human Factors. *Quality in Health Care*, Vol. 4: 80–89.

Reason, J., A. Manstead, S. Stradling, J. Baxter, and K. Campbell. (1990). Errors and Violations on the Roads: A Real Distinction? *Ergonomics* Vol. 33, No. 10–11: 1315–1332.

Rice, R. S., and F. Dell'Amico. (1974). An Experimental Study of Automobile Driver Characteristics and Capabilities. CALSPAN-ZS-5208-K-1. Calspan Corporation, Buffalo, NY.

Richard, C. M., and M. G. Lichty. (2013). Driver Expectations When Navigating Complex Interchanges. FHWA-HRT-13-048. U.S. Department of Transportation, Federal Highway Administration, Washington, DC.

Richard, C. M., J. L. Campbell, and J. L. Brown. (2006). Task Analysis of Intersection Driving Scenarios: Information Processing Bottlenecks. FHWA-HRT-06-033. U.S. Department of Transportation, Federal Highway Administration, Washington, DC.

Richard, C. M., K. Magee, P. Bacon-Abdelmoteleb, and J. L. Brown. (2018). Countermeasures that Work: A Highway Safety Countermeasure Guide for State Highway Safety Offices, Ninth Edition. DOT HS 812 478. U.S. Department of Transportation, National Highway Traffic Safety Administration, Washington, DC.

Roadway Safety Foundation. (2024a). What is usRAP? United States Road Assessment Program, Washington, DC. http://www.usrap.org/what-usrap.

Roadway Safety Foundation. (2024b). Who Should Use usRAP? United States Road Assessment Program, Washington, DC. www.usrap.org/who-should-use-usrap.

Russell, E. R. (1998). Using Concepts of Driver Expectancy, Positive Guidance and Consistency for Improved Operation and Safety. *1998 Transportation Conference Proceedings*.

Sando, T., and W. Hunter. (2014). Operational Analysis of Shared Lane Markings and Green Bike Lanes on Roadways with Speeds Greater than 35 Mph. BDK82-977-04. Florida Department of Transportation, Tallahassee, FL.

Shafer, M. A. (1996). Driver Mental Workload Requirements on Horizontal Curves Based on Occluded Vision Test Measurements. TTI-04690-2. Texas Transportation Institute, College Station, TX.

Signor, K., W. Kumfer, S. LaJeunesse, D. Carter, W. Smith, M. Scaringelli, and S. Deans. (2018). Safe Systems Synthesis: An International Scan for Domestic Application. UNC Highway Safety Research Center, Chapel Hill, NC.

Singh, S. (2015). Critical Reasons for Crashes Investigated in the National Motor Vehicle Crash Causation Survey. Traffic Safety Facts Crash Statistics Report No. DOT HS 812 506. U.S. Department of Transportation, National Highway Traffic Safety Administration, Washington, DC.

Stuster, J. (2019). Task Analysis: How to Develop an Understanding of Work. Human Factors and Ergonomics Society, Washington, DC.

Stuster, J., and R. Roesch. (2001). Salient Human Factors Issues Concerning the Landing Craft Air Cushion (LCAC). Technical Report for Naval Coastal Systems Station, Anacapa Sciences, Inc., Panama City, FL.

Summala, H. (1981). Drivers' Steering Reaction to a Light Stimulus on a Dark Road. *Ergonomics* Vol. 24, No. 2: 125–131.

Theeuwes, J. (2021). Self-Explaining Roads: What Does Visual Cognition Tell Us About Designing Safer Roads? *Cognitive Research: Principles and Implications*, Vol. 6: 1–15.

Theeuwes, J., and R. van der Horst. (2012). *Designing Safe Road Systems: A Human Factors Perspective*. CRC Press, Boca Raton, FL.

Tignor, S. C. (2022). Quantification Metrics and Analysis of Human Factor, Workload, and Road Infrastructure. *Transportation Research Record: Journal of the Transportation Research Board*, No. 2676: 773–784. https://doi.org/10.1177/03611981211033860.

Tignor, S. C. (2023). Enhancing Highway Functional Classifications with Road User Demands. *Transportation Research Record: Journal of the Transportation Research Board*, No. 2677: 284–294. https://doi.org/10.1177/03611981231168102.

Tijerina, L., N. Browning, S. J. Mangold, E. F. Madigan, and J. A. Pierowicz. (1995a). Examination of Reduced Visibility Crashes and Potential IVHS Countermeasures. DOT HS 808 201. U.S. Department of Transportation, National Highway Traffic Safety Administration, Washington, DC.

Tijerina, L., B. H. Kantowitz, S. M. Kiger, and T. H. Rockwell. (1995b). Driver Workload Assessment of In-Cab High Technology Devices. *Proceedings: International Technical Conference on the Enhanced Safety of Vehicles*, Vol. 1995: 330–342. U.S. Department of Transportation, National Highway Traffic Safety Administration, Washington, DC.

Tijerina, L., S. Kiger, T. Rockwell, C. Tornow, J. Kinateder, and F. Kokkotos. (1996). Heavy Vehicle Driver Workload Assessment. Task 6, Baseline Data Study. DOT HS-808 467. U.S. Department of Transportation, National Highway Traffic Safety Administration, Washington, DC.

Tijerina, L., F. S. Barickman, and E. N. Mazzae. (2004). Driver Eye Glance Behavior During Car Following. DOT-HS-809-723. U.S. Department of Transportation, National Highway Traffic Safety Administration, Washington, DC.

Tivesten, E., and M. Dozza. (2015). Driving Context Influences Drivers' Decision to Engage in Visual-Manual Phone Tasks: Evidence from a Naturalistic Driving Study. *Journal of Safety Research*, Vol. 53: 87–96.

Torbic, D. J., K. M. Bauer, C. A. Fees, D. W. Harwood, R. Van Houten, J. LaPlante, and N. Roseberry. (2014). *NCHRP Report 766: Recommended Bicycle Lane Widths for Various Roadway Characteristics*. Transportation Research Board of the National Academies, Washington, DC.

Treat, J. R., N. S. Tumbas, S. T. McDonald, D. Shinar, and R. D. Hume. (1979). Tri-Level Study of the Causes of Traffic Accidents, Executive Summary. DOTHS034353579TAC [5]. U.S. Department of Transportation, National Highway Traffic Safety Administration, Washington, DC.

Triggs, T. J., and W. G. Harris. (1982). Reaction Time of Drivers to Road Stimuli. Human Factors Report No. HFR-12. Monash University, Melbourne, Australia.

Tsyganov, A., R. Machemehl, and R. Harrison. (2002). Complex Work Zone Safety. FHWA/TX-03/4021-3. Texas Department of Transportation, Austin, TX.

Turanski, A., and L. Tijerina. (1996). Heavy Vehicle Driver Workload Assessment–Task 2: Standard Vehicle Configuration/Task Specifications. DOT HS 808 467 [2]. U.S. Department of Transportation, National Highway Traffic Safety Administration, Washington, DC. https://rosap.ntl.bts.gov/view/dot/4058.

United States Army. (2014). Human Systems Integration. United States Army. https://www.army.mil/standto/archive/2014/12/17/.

Venkatraman, V., C. M. Richard, K. Magee, and K. Johnson. (2021). Countermeasures That Work: A Highway Safety Countermeasures Guide for State Highway Safety Offices. DOT HS 813 097. U.S. Department of Transportation, National Highway Traffic Safety Administration, Washington, DC.

Victor, T., M. Dozza, J. Bärgman, C. N. Boda, J. Engström, C. Flannagan, J. D. Lee, and G. Markkula. (2015). *Analysis of Naturalistic Driving Study Data: Safer Glances, Driver Inattention, and Crash Risk*. SHRP 2 Report S2-S08A-RW-1. Strategic Highway Research Program, Transportation Research Board, Washington, DC.

Washington State Department of Licensing (WDL). (2022). Commercial Driver Guide. Olympia, WA. https://driving-tests.org/washington/wa-cdl-handbook/.

Welle, B., A. B. Sharpin, C. Adriazola-Steil, S. Alveano, M. Obelheiro, C. T. Imamoglu, S. Job, M. Shotten, and D. Bose. (2018). Sustainable and Safe: A Vision and Guidance for Zero Road Deaths. World Resources Institute, Washington, DC.

Wickens, C. D. (1992). *Engineering Psychology and Human Performance*. Harper Collins, New York, NY.

Wickens, C. D. (2008). Multiple Resources and Mental Workload. *Human Factors: The Journal of the Human Factors and Ergonomics Society*, Vol. 50: 449–455.

Wierwille, W. W., R. J. Hanowski, J. M. Hankey, C. A. Kieliszewski, S. E. Lee, A. Medina, A. S. Keisler, and T. A. Dingus. (2002). Identification and Evaluation of Driver Errors: Overview and Recommendations. FHWA-RD-02-003. U.S. Department of Transportation, Federal Highway Administration, Washington, DC.

Williams, K., V. G. Stover, K. Dixon, and P. Demosthenes. (2014). *Access Management Manual, Second Edition*. Transportation Research Board, Washington, DC.

Wilson, E. M., and M. E. Lipinski. (2004). *NCHRP Synthesis 336: Road Safety Audits*. Transportation Research Board of the National Academies, Washington, DC.

Xie, L., C. Wu, N. Lyu, and Z. Duan. (2019). Studying the Effects of Freeway Alignment, Traffic Flow, and Sign Information on Subjective Driving Workload and Performance. *Advances in Mechanical Engineering*, Vol. 11, No. 5: 1687814019853690.

Zegeer, C., R. Srinivasan, B. Lan, D. Carter, S. Smith, C. Sundstrom, N. Thirsk, C. Lyon, B. Persaud, J. Zegeer, E. Ferguson, and R. Van Houten. (2017). *NCHRP Research Report 841: Development of Crash Modification Factors for Uncontrolled Pedestrian Crossing Treatments*. Transportation Research Board, Washington, DC.

Acronyms and Abbreviations

BAC	Blood alcohol content
BTSCRP	Behavioral Traffic Safety Cooperative Research Program
CMF	Crash modification factors
DOT	Department of transportation
EMS	Emergency medical services
FARS	Fatality Analysis Reporting System
FHWA	Federal Highway Administration
HFG	Human Factors Guidelines
HFIM	Human Factors Interaction Matrix
HSIP	Highway Safety Improvement Program
HSM	Highway Safety Manual
IHSDM	Interactive Highway Safety Design Model
MMI	Most meaningful information
MUTCD	Manual on Uniform Traffic Control Devices
NACTO	National Association of City Transportation Officials
NCHRP	National Cooperative Highway Research Program
NCSA	National Center for Statistics and Analysis
NDS	Naturalistic driving study
NHTSA	National Highway Traffic Safety Administration
NMVCCS	National Motor Vehicle Crash Causation Survey
NTSB	National Transportation Safety Board
PDO	Property damage only
PIARC	Permanent International Association of Road Congresses
PPE	Personal protective equipment
PRT	Perception-response time
RSA	Road Safety Audit
RSAR	Road Safety Audit Review
SHSP	Strategic Highway Safety Plans
SHRP 2	Strategic Highway Research Program 2
SPF	Safety performance function
TAWL	Task Analysis/Workload
TSM&O	Transportation Systems Management and Operations
usRAP	United States Road Assessment Program
VRU	Vulnerable road users

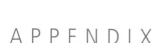

Summary of Current Diagnostic Assessment and Countermeasure Selection Tools for Crashes

1 Introduction

This subsection reviews diagnostic assessments and countermeasure selection approaches used to assess and mitigate roadway crashes. This is a substantial field, and the goal was not to capture every instance of these methodologies; rather, it was to generally present the breadth and nature of the current state of the art of diagnostic assessment and countermeasure selection. The following resources are presented and described as follows:

- Program Evaluation

- *Highway Safety Manual* (HSM)

- usRAP (Roadway Safety Foundation, 2024b)

- Systemic Safety Project Selection Tool

- Safe System

- PEDSAFE (FHWA, n.d.c) and BIKESAFE (FHWA, n.d.a)

- *Field Guide for Selecting Countermeasures at Uncontrolled Pedestrian Crossing Locations* (Blackburn et al., 2018)

- Use of naturalistic driving study (NDS) data

2 Program Evaluation

State highway safety plans (e.g., SHSPs) use safety data—such as fatal crashes and crashes involving serious injuries along with roadway and traffic data—to identify critical highway safety problems and safety improvement opportunities. These plans include specific multi-year goals, objectives, and measures to support performance-based highway programs. Specific strategies for improving safety include the highway safety elements of engineering, education, enforcement, and emergency services (the four "E's"; FHWA, 2016).

From FHWA (2016): "For example, if speed is an emphasis area in a State SHSP, the State may consider a variety of 4 E strategies to reduce or mitigate the impact of speeding. Strategies might include increasing law enforcement efforts to reduce speeding (enforcement), applying traffic calming measures such as speed humps and roundabouts (engineering), delivering public information campaigns that focus on the dangers of speeding (education), and utilizing Emergency Medical Services data to quantify the burden to the health care system and the cost to the community (emergency services)."

Equally critical to improving safety performance is the evaluation (the fifth "E" of safety) of crash data in modal and facility contexts to assess and aid the selection and design of countermeasures. While program evaluation might be considered something to worry about after countermeasures have been identified, this fifth "E" should be implemented at every stage of the safety improvement process (see Figure 1) and include input and involvement from the range of transportation professionals involved, including planners, designers, engineers, and safety analysts. In short, having an evaluative mindset throughout the crash prevention process can add rigor and purpose to safety improvement planning.
Evaluation is simply the process of examining the value or worth of something. In the highway safety context, evaluations focus on rigorously analyzing and assessing the efficacy of safety improvements to determine what is working and why. As described in Pullen-Seufert and Hall (2008), evaluations should be seen as a tool to be used throughout the highway safety improvement process to clarify problems, help develop good safety questions, prioritize countermeasures, identify metrics for success, and then assess countermeasure implementations. At its most fundamental level, countermeasure evaluations focus on two basic questions: (1) did you implement the program as planned? and (2) did you accomplish your objectives? (Pullen-Seufert and Hall, 2008).

Pullen-Seufert and Hall (2008) provide a seven-step process for evaluating highway safety programs and countermeasures, as follows:

1. **Identify the problem:** Gather and analyze the information necessary to help determine the nature and size of the problem you wish to address, data on contributing factors, where the problem is manifesting, and who is being affected.

2. **Develop reasonable objectives:** What will determine the success of a proposed program, treatment, or countermeasure, and how will success be measured? Program objectives should be SMART (specific, measurable, action-oriented, reasonable, and time-specific) (Pullen-Seufert and Hall, 2008).

3. **Develop a plan for measuring results:** Develop a detailed plan that describes what you will measure, how you will measure it, and how you will analyze the results obtained. In general, evaluations are more robust when they include multiple measures obtained from multiple methods—it is beneficial to consider a range of outcome measures that are appropriate to your evaluations. For example, a countermeasure to reduce speeding behavior might use speeding-involved crashes, speeding tickets, and surveys of public awareness to assess efficacy.

4. **Gather baseline data:** Measuring the value of a proposed program, treatment, or countermeasure often includes comparing measured outcomes before implementation to those same outcomes after implementation, while controlling for other key variables that could impact the results.

5. **Implement your program:** Initiate the program, treatment, or countermeasure that is the focus of your evaluation and document all implementation issues, questions, or milestones that might be important as you analyze your data.

6. **Gather data and analyze results:** Data collection and analysis may well be the most complex and labor-intensive elements of an evaluation. In this regard, a data collection schedule with detailed procedures should be developed and followed. Pay close attention to any external events that could change your outcomes in ways that are separate from the program, treatment, or countermeasure under evaluation. For example, if you are monitoring the effects of a countermeasure to reduce speeding behavior through a specific section of roadway and that roadway undergoes a major revision involving work zones and reduced traffic and throughput, you may wish to delay the evaluation or shift the implementation to another roadway to avoid confounding the results.

7. **Report results:** Clearly communicate the objectives, methods, results and conclusions of your evaluation to all organizations involved in the effort.

3   Highway Safety Manual

The American Association of State Highway and Transportation Officials (AASHTO) HSM is a resource that provides safety knowledge and tools in a useful form to facilitate improved decision-making based on safety performance (AASHTO, 2010). The six steps of the roadway safety management process are presented in Figure 1 in this appendix and are described in this section. The inputs and outputs for each step vary based on the safety management approach employed. The six-step roadway safety management process helps agencies develop a prioritized list of safety improvement projects and then evaluate the effectiveness of the projects in reducing crash frequency and/or severity.

1. **Network Screening**—Review a transportation network to identify and rank individual sites based on the potential for reducing crashes.

2. **Diagnosis**—Evaluate crash data, historic site data, and field conditions to identify crash patterns of interest at each site.

3. **Countermeasure Selection**—Identify factors that may contribute to crashes at a site and select possible countermeasures to reduce crashes.

4. **Economic Appraisal**—Calculate the estimated benefits and costs of potential countermeasures and identify individual projects that are cost-effective or economically justified.

5. **Project Prioritization**—Evaluate economically justified improvements at specific sites and across sites to identify a set of improvement projects that meet objectives such as cost, mobility, or environmental impacts.

6. **Safety Effectiveness Evaluation**—Evaluate the effectiveness of a countermeasure, a combination of countermeasures, or projects implemented at multiple sites in reducing crash frequency and/or severity.

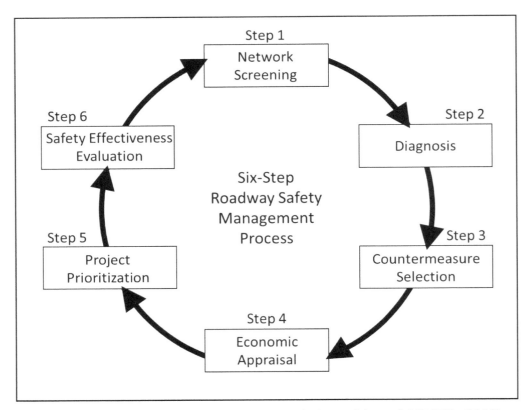

Figure 1.   Six-step safety management process (adapted from AASHTO, 2010).

The roadway safety management process may be conducted sequentially as described, or each step may be conducted in isolation. This project focused on Steps 2 and 3 of the roadway safety management process. As noted above, however, the fifth E—evaluation—should be applied throughout the entire process.

The three primary steps associated with diagnosis outlined in the HSM are as follows (AASHTO, 2010):

1. Review safety data such as crash types, severities, and environmental conditions to develop descriptive statistics and identify crash patterns.

2. Review supporting documentation, such as past studies and plans covering the site vicinity, to identify known issues, opportunities, and constraints.

3. Conduct a field investigation to assess the conditions of the site and observe how different users and modes travel through the site and use available facilities and services in the vicinity of the site.

The HSM describes the three primary steps of countermeasure selection (AASHTO, 2010):

1. Identify factors contributing to the cause of crashes at the subject site.

2. Identify countermeasures that may address the contributing factors.

3. Conduct a cost-benefit analysis, if possible, to select preferred treatments.

Although the HSM has several different types of documentation—including user guides—to assist with understanding the approach, the tools may be difficult for some to navigate. For example, the diagnostic process includes human factors as an integral component of its procedure; however, the HSM lacks a systematic and fully guided approach to human factors insofar as there does not exist a checklist or set of detailed diagnostic questions related to specific human factors issues. Such a tool that maintains a level of specificity would be beneficial. Rather than relying on the users to understand what features fall under each human factors category, users will be able to simply be guided by the tool itself.

4   usRAP

The usRAP is a free and proactive safety management tool used to rate the safety of a roadway based on an assessment of the presence and condition of the roadway, roadside, and intersection design elements and to identify cost-effective countermeasures to reduce fatal and serious injury crashes (Roadway Safety Foundation, 2024b). This tool is used by state and local highway agencies, and each agency's data are password protected. The usRAP is not meant to take the place of professional engineering studies, RSAs, or other activities carried out by roadway agencies and traffic engineers; but, this data-driven tool provides proactive procedures to assess crash potential, mapping capabilities, and cost-benefit considerations to identify cost-effective countermeasures to reduce fatal and serious injury crashes (Roadway Safety Foundation, 2024a).

Data for roadway networks are collected and inputted into a software package that assigns a star rating (from one to five), reflecting the socioeconomic cost of crashes on the particular road section. The data needed for the software may be acquired from existing highway agency databases. When these data are unavailable, the required data input may be coded from Internet-based roadway photos or video logs.

The tool can be used to perform two types of analysis: developing star ratings and developing safer road investment plans. Star ratings and safer road investment plans are developed for 328-ft (100-m) sections of roadway, combined to provide recommended improvements for specific road sections, entire routes, and entire road networks.

Star ratings provide insight into crash likelihood and crash protection. Star ratings are based on the presence or absence of design and traffic control features associated with safety on an area of a roadway. A rating of one star indicates a road has few safety-related design and traffic features, whereas a rating of five indicates a road has many safety-related design and traffic features. Separate star ratings are provided for vehicle occupants, bicyclists, pedestrians, and motorcyclists because features that affect crash frequencies for these different modes of travel are very different.

After star ratings are assigned, the software evaluates approximately 70 countermeasures for potential implementation. If there appears to be an engineering need for a countermeasure and that countermeasure is not already present on the roadway segment, the countermeasure is identified for consideration in an economic analysis, and the software performs a cost-benefit analysis for every countermeasure that was identified during the process. This output is referred to as a safer roads investment plan. Although site-specific crash data are not required, crash data are highly recommended for appropriate calibration to local conditions. The safer roads investment plan considers estimates of how many lives could be saved over 20 years if each improvement specified by the plan was made.

According to the usRAP website, this tool is user-friendly in that it does not require extensive crash data and, instead, uses aerial photos or video logs and free online software to generate a safer road investment plan (Roadway Safety Foundation, 2024a). Furthermore, the usRAP protocols and video software are available for free. The usRAP trainings may also be accessed free of charge. However, acquiring all of the required elements to utilize usRAP may be time-consuming. Additionally, the mention of human factors is absent from their website and other associated documentation. The software selects the use of potential countermeasures automatically without taking into consideration contributing factors of the crashes.

5   Systemic Safety Project Selection Tool

The Systemic Safety Project Selection Tool is used by state and local highway agencies and transportation planning organizations (Preston et al., 2013). The aim is to assist agencies with performing a systemwide evaluation—rather than site-specific analyses—to identify roadway features common to locations with a crash history; this process enables agencies to proactively address crashes that are widely dispersed across a highway and is considered more beneficial for countermeasure development versus diagnosing individual crashes (Preston et al., 2013).

Similar to the HSM, this tool presents a cyclical safety management process that involves three elements:

1. **The Systemic Safety Planning Process** helps analysts identify priority crash types and associated crash contributing factors, evaluate proven, low-cost safety countermeasures, and prioritize candidate locations for improvement.

2. **A Framework for Balancing Systemic and Traditional Safety Investments** that helps set funding goals between systemic and traditional safety programs.

3. **Program Evaluation Methods** that provide high-level direction for evaluating the effectiveness of systemic safety programs.

Of the three elements, the systemic safety planning process addresses diagnosis and countermeasure selection at various levels. The systemic safety planning process begins by identifying focus crash types, facility types, and contributing factors. The next steps involve documenting and/or identifying the most common characteristics of the locations where each focus crash type occurred and developing a prioritized list of potential locations on the roadway system that could benefit from systemic safety improvement projects. The data required to establish this include observations of site-specific crash information and basic features of the road system. Once facility types are identified, the factors contributing to roadway crashes along the network and at specific locations are assessed. The outcome of this process is an assessment and ranking of the focus facility elements in terms of their priority for safety improvement. The next stage of the safety planning process involves assembling a list of potential countermeasures, screening and evaluating said countermeasures, and selecting the countermeasures for deployment. This step involves assembling a small number of low-cost, highly effective countermeasures to be considered for project development at candidate locations.

Overall, this diagnostic tool is flexible (applicable to various systems, locations, and crash types), easy to use (requires minimal training and assistance), and easy to understand (the output is understandable by program managers and development engineers). Regarding the steps involving diagnosis and countermeasure selection, little guidance is provided in terms of how to select countermeasures to address the crash-contributing factors. In addition, the inclusion of human factors is minimal, as this tool only tends to mention poor visibility and excessive speed as potential crash-contributing factors (Preston et al., 2013).

6   Safe System

The Safe System approach is a worldwide movement implemented since the 1990s (Signor et al., 2018; Welle et al., 2018) via programs such as Vision Zero in Sweden and other countries. According to the Federal Highway Administration (FHWA), the Safe System approach is one way to reduce deaths and serious injuries on the road (Welle et al., 2018; Finkel et al., 2020). The World Health Organization has expressed a similar perspective of the approach, but with a particular emphasis on human involvement, as it has stated that the goal of Safe System is to ensure that if crashes occur, humans are not seriously injured (Finkel et al., 2020).

The Safe System approach has been claimed to encompass an interaction of issues that lead to roadway deaths and injuries; that is, it prioritizes the protection of VRUs (e.g., pedestrians and cyclists) and emphasizes the responsibility of roadway system designers (Welle et al., 2018). For example, the Safe System approach would contend that humans make mistakes and are fragile and vulnerable. Consequently—to address roadway issues—one aim of a Safe System approach would be to reduce the need and length of driving trips (Finkel et al., 2020). Furthermore, Safe System emphasizes the importance of designing and operating transportation systems that are "human-centric" and accommodate such vulnerabilities (e.g., managing kinetic energy transfer within survivable limits to inform the design and operation of the road system).

The areas that Safe System focuses on are motivated by six core principles (Signor et al., 2018; Welle et al., 2018; Finkel et al., 2020):

1. Death/serious injury is unacceptable.

2. Humans make mistakes/errors.

3. Humans are vulnerable to injury.

4. Safety is proactive.

5. Responsibility is shared.

6. Redundancy is crucial.

As a result of these motivating principles, the Safe System approach aims to integrate five elements to promote a safe transportation system, the first of which is safe road users who comply with the rules of the road. Compliance is demonstrated by behaviors such as paying attention and adapting to changing conditions. The second is having safe vehicles on the road that are equipped with appropriate safety features (e.g., airbags, seatbelts) and an effective design. Others include promoting safe speeds and roads and the final deals with post-crash care (e.g., providing emergency services and crash/reporting investigation) (Finkel et al., 2020).

In addition to promoting the importance of the human in the process of enhancing roadway safety, the Safe System approach also emphasizes several other factors that are purportedly integral to mitigating issues on the road. One such factor is that responsibility is shared by various stakeholders (e.g., road users and system managers), who work together to provide safety countermeasures (Finkel et al., 2020). Furthermore, the approach underscores proactive tools to identify and mitigate crash potential on the roadway system and redundancy so that if something fails, there will exist other parts to mitigate crash potential (Finkel et al., 2020). These factors interact with human factors, such as, for example, implementing redundancy via rumble strips to alert a drowsy or distracted driver (Finkel et al., 2020). There still exists, however, a lack of clear attention on human factors, such as visibility and time perception, and clear, actionable items or strategies that may be utilized to directly target a wide variety of human factors characteristics. Indeed, it is clear that more attention must be focused on bridging the gap between theoretical strategies implied by the Safe System approach and current practices.

7   PEDSAFE and BIKESAFE

PEDSAFE (FHWA, n.d.c) and BIKESAFE (FHWA, n.d.a) are intended primarily for use by engineers, planners, safety professionals, and decision-makers, but they may also be used by citizens for identifying problems and recommending solutions for their communities associated with walking and biking. PEDSAFE and BIKESAFE are online tools intended to provide the most applicable information for identifying safety and mobility needs and improving conditions for pedestrians and bicyclists within the public right-of-way. These tools are designed to enable practitioners to select engineering, education, and enforcement countermeasures to help mitigate known crash problems and/or to help achieve a specific performance objective. The tools

- Provide information about pedestrian and bicycle crash types, statistics, and other background resources;

- Provide users with information on what countermeasures are available to prevent specific categories of pedestrian and bicycle crashes or to achieve certain performance objectives;

- Outline considerations to be addressed in the selection of a countermeasure;

- Provide a decision process to eliminate countermeasures from the list of possibilities; and

- Provide case studies of countermeasures introduced in communities throughout the United States.

These tools have several options for selecting potential countermeasures. There is an interactive selection tool that allows the user to develop a list of possible countermeasures based on site characteristics, such as geometric features and operating conditions and the type of safety problem or desired behavioral change. The user first inputs information about the location of the site. Then, the user must decide on the goal of the treatment. It may either be to achieve a specific performance objective, such as reducing traffic volumes or mitigating a specific type of pedestrian/bicycle collision. Once a specific goal has been selected, the analyst provides answers to a series of questions related to the geometric and operational characteristics of the site. The answers are used to narrow the list of appropriate countermeasures for a specific goal.

Another option for selecting potential countermeasures is through the use of interactive matrices that provide the user with a quick view of the relationship between performance objectives and several countermeasure groups or the relationships between several crash types and countermeasure groups. In either matrix, a filled cell indicates that there is a specific countermeasure within the countermeasure group, this applies to the performance objectives or crash types. From there, the analyst can choose to select a countermeasure and be linked to the countermeasure description.

Overall, these tools are easy to use and accessible online via the FHWA's Pedestrian Safety Guide and Countermeasure Selection System (PEDSAFE) (FHWA, n.d.c). These tools are also incorporated in the Pedestrian and Bicycle Crash Analysis Tool (FHWA, 2023c). With each countermeasure included in the tools, a description of the treatment is provided along with its purpose, other considerations that one should be aware of, and cost estimates. The inclusion of human factors considerations is minimal.

7.1   Guide for Selecting Countermeasures at Uncontrolled Crossing Locations

The *Field Guide for Selecting Countermeasures at Uncontrolled Pedestrian Crossing Locations* (Blackburn et al., 2018) helps agencies select crash countermeasures based on criteria established in published literature, best practices, and national guidance. The tool describes a comprehensive decision-making process for the installation of pedestrian crossing countermeasures and leads an agency through the process. The steps involve

- Collecting data and engaging the public,

- Collecting an inventory of the site conditions and prioritizing locations,

- Analyzing crash types and safety issues,

- Selecting countermeasures,

- Consulting design and installation resources, and

- Identifying opportunities and monitoring outcomes.

The tool focuses on selecting countermeasures at uncontrolled crossing locations—where sidewalks or designated walkways intersect a roadway where no traffic control (i.e., traffic signal or stop sign) is present. The countermeasures described in the tool include

- Crosswalk visibility enhancements,

- Raised crosswalks,

- Pedestrian refuge islands,

- Pedestrian hybrid beacons, and

- Road diets.

The *Field Guide for Selecting Countermeasures at Uncontrolled Pedestrian Crossing Locations* (Blackburn et al., 2018) describes each countermeasure and presents additional design and installation considerations, such as references to the *Manual on Uniform Traffic Control Devices* (MUTCD) (FHWA, 2009).

This tool presents two tables for a practitioner to identify potential countermeasures. The first table (Application of Pedestrian Crash Countermeasures by Roadway Feature) identifies suggested countermeasures for uncontrolled crossing locations according to roadway and traffic features. Features addressed in the table include the number of lanes, median type, speed limit, and traffic volumes. The second table (Safety Issues Addressed per Countermeasure) compares crash types and other observed safety issues to the countermeasures. The safety issues addressed within this table include conflicts at crossing locations, excessive vehicle speed, inadequate conspicuity/visibility, drivers not yielding to pedestrians in crosswalks, and insufficient separation from traffic.

The *Field Guide for Selecting Countermeasures at Uncontrolled Pedestrian Crossing Locations* is relatively simple to use. A field guide is available that provides instructions on how to use the tables and a sample inventory form for agencies to record information about roadway characteristics, and safety issues and descriptions of the countermeasures are provided.

7.2   Use of Naturalistic Driving Study Data

NDSs offer great potential to help identify and prioritize contributing factors to crashes, and for supporting countermeasure development and assessments; to date, such studies have been extremely valuable in clarifying how driver performance and behavior affect the potential of roadway crashes (Victor et al., 2015). One such study is the 100-Car NDS sponsored by the NHTSA and the Virginia Department of Transportation (Dingus et al., 2006). According to Dingus et al. (2006), the "100-Car Naturalistic Driving Study is the first instrumented vehicle study undertaken with the primary purpose of collecting large-scale naturalistic driving data" (p. xxii). The NDS was unobtrusive in that participants were asked to freely drive as they typically would, thereby creating a database of naturalistic driver behaviors, such as aggressive driving, drowsiness, judgment error, and so forth (Dingus et al., 2006). Additionally, the naturalistic nature of the study provides information about pre-crash and crash events that are externally valid (Dingus et al., 2006).

Indeed, in a report that conducted analyses of driver inattention using the driving data that were collected from the 100-Cars NDS, the results revealed that driving while drowsy led to a higher probability of a near-crash/crash risk compared to alert drivers and that drivers who engage in visually and/or manually complex tasks also have a higher probability of near-crash/crash risk than those who are attentive (Klauer et al., 2006). Not only did the NDS data reveal human factors that increase near-crash/crash risk, but it also clarified environmental factors that heighten the probability of such risk. For instance, the data showed that driving while drowsy is more dangerous when passing through intersections, wet roadways, and high-traffic areas (Klauer et al., 2006). NDSs have also revealed how driving context influences a driver's decision to partake in visual-manual phone tasks (i.e., texting, dialing, reading) (Tivesten and Dozza, 2015).

As a further example, consider the problem of red-light running at intersections. One cause of red-light running occurs when drivers have difficulty deciding whether to stop at the stop line or proceed through the intersection as they approach a traffic signal that recently changed from green to yellow. Often in this situation, a "dilemma zone" is created if the vehicle is too close to stop safely before the stop-line but too far away to clear the intersection before the signal changes to red (for a more detailed discussion of the dilemma zone, see Campbell et al., 2012). A wide range of situational factors affects driver behavior in a dilemma zone situation and red-light running. In dilemma zones, these include factors such as yellow duration, cycle length, surrounding vehicle actions, approach speed, driver age, and gender, among several other factors. Yet, approaches for calculating dilemma zones typically only include basic variables such as vehicle speed measures, distance, and driver response time. While the concept of the dilemma zone is relatively simple and is often treated as such, the environmental, situational, and driver aspects underlying the decision to stop or run a yellow/red light are substantially more complex. NDS data, such as data obtained from the Strategic Highway Research Program 2 (SHRP 2) (AASHTO, n.d.a) can provide answers to the following questions:

1. What are the circumstances surrounding red-light running, and what immediate situational factors (e.g., roadside distraction, lead vehicle going, high pedestrian traffic volume, and so forth) are associated with this behavior?

2. What is the relationship between the calculated dilemma zone for an intersection and what drivers actually do? What driver, situational, location-specific, and environment factors (see Table 1) are associated with drivers, making them lead to crashes or increased crash potential? How do these driver decisions/actions vary across intersections with different characteristics?

3. How do drivers respond to dilemma zone situations? What factors incline drivers to stop or to go at yellow onset (e.g., signal timing, signal visibility, driver attention, and so forth)?

Specifically, NDS data like the SHRP 2 data provide a unique opportunity to examine driver red-light running and dilemma zone behavior by providing a detailed picture of the driving situation and driver actions leading up to an intersection immediately before the traffic signal changes, including several types of data that can be extracted from the SHRP 2 driving and roadway data files (see Table 1).

Table 1. **Variables from the SHRP 2 data set relevant to studying dilemma zone behaviors.**

Type	Variable
Vehicle	Vehicle type, distance from the intersection, speed, acceleration/deceleration level, lead vehicle present, familiar/unfamiliar driver
Driver behavior	Accelerator and/or brake presses, general eye-glance location, eyes-off road, facial expression
Traffic	Signal status, presence and leading and following vehicles, actions of vehicles in adjacent lanes, time waiting at the intersection
Environment	Time-of-day/ambient light, weather conditions, presence of pedestrians and bikes, traffic signal occlusion by other trucks
Site Characteristics	Signal timing, number of lanes, lane width, presence of bicycle facilities, traffic volume, signal type/visibility, roadside distractions, historical pedestrian use levels

A particularly valuable feature of the SHRP 2 NDS data is that the listed variables are generally available for each traversal of an intersection, which provides an opportunity to take a comprehensive and holistic look at driver behaviors in dilemma zones, in contrast to the other studies that typically only examine a small number of these variables at a time. Taken together, these examples demonstrate how NDS data can elucidate particular human and environmental factors that influence roadway crash risk and, therefore, have implications for which areas to consider when developing diagnostic and countermeasure resources.